GASTROENTEROLOGY

for kids

Medical
School
FOR KIDS™

First paperback edition June 2022

Book design by Betty Nguyen & Brandon Pham

ISBN 978-1-957557-04-5 (paperback)

Printed in the United States of America

Published by Black Phoenix Press

www.mdforkids.org

Disclaimer: Contents of this book are for informational purposes only. No material in this book is intended to provide, or be a substitute for, professional medical advice.

To the friends and family who have supported and loved us unconditionally, and to the mentors who have guided and taught us more than we could have imagined:

Thank you.

Betty & Brandon

Medical School FOR KIDS™

Gastroenterology

(ga-strow-en-ter-AH-luh-jee)

the branch of medicine concerned with the study and treatment of disorders of the stomach and intestines

Medical School FOR KIDS™

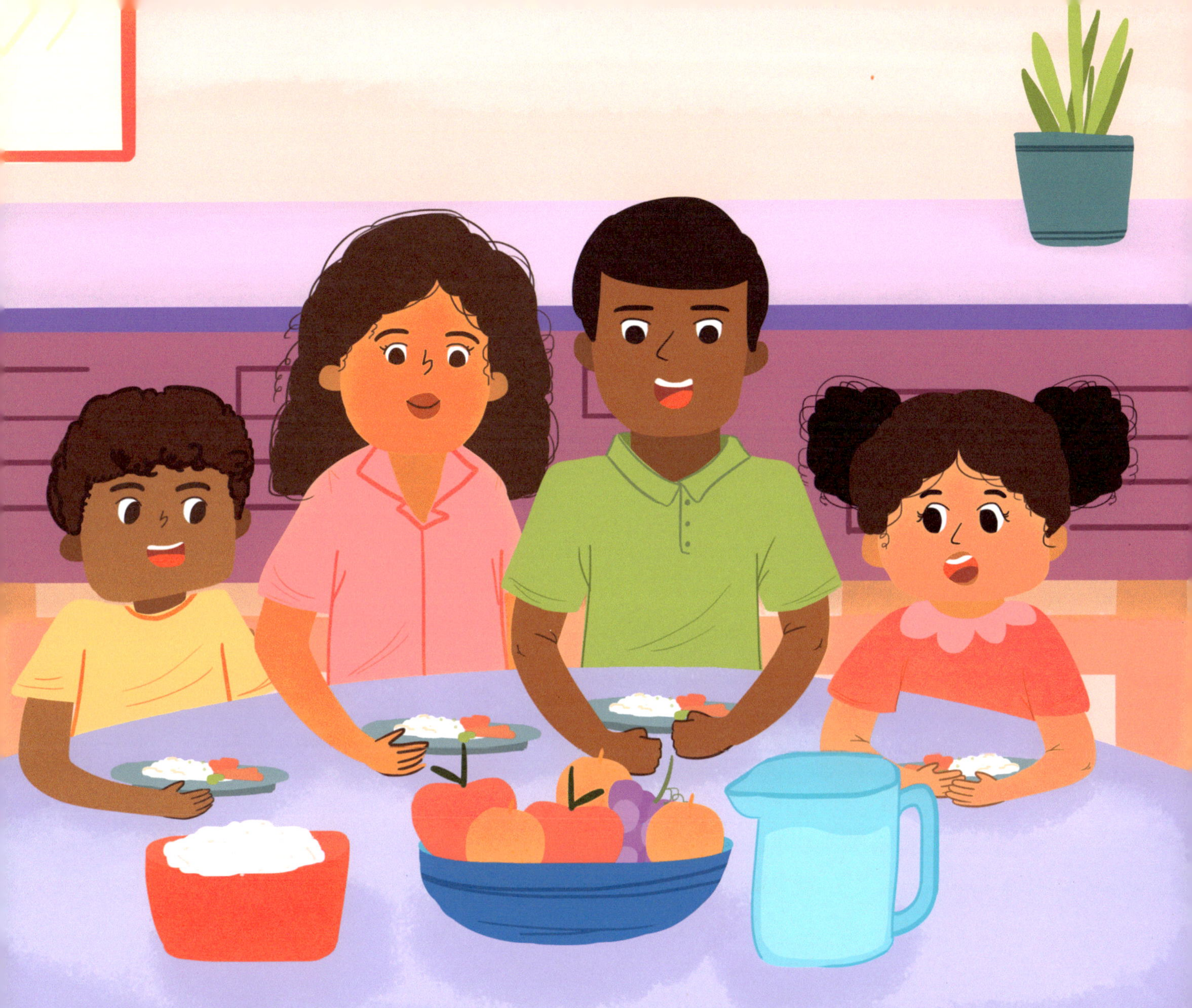

We all need to eat food to survive.
Where does food go after we eat it?

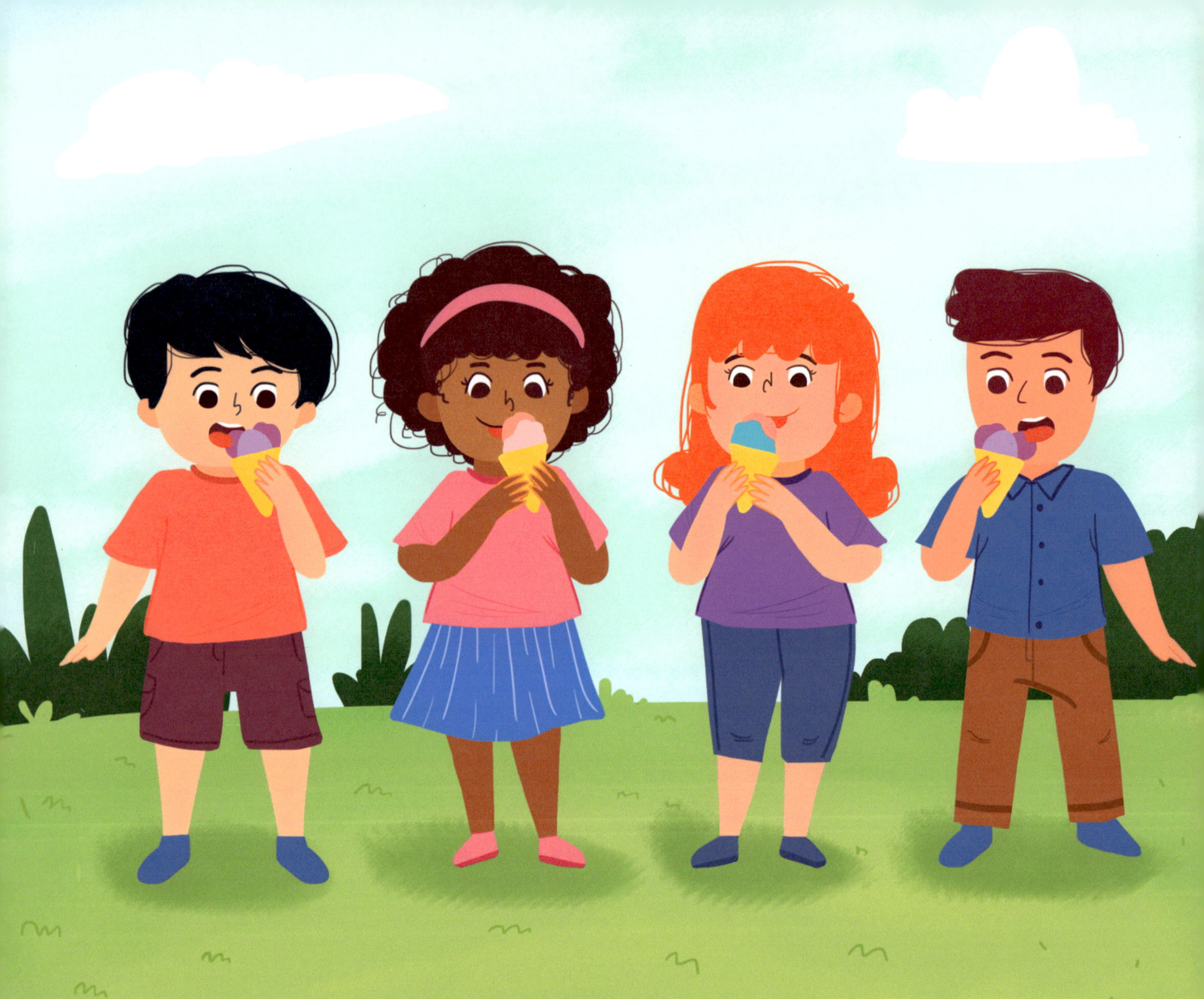

First, food goes into our mouth. Our **tongue** allows us to taste food. Yum yum!

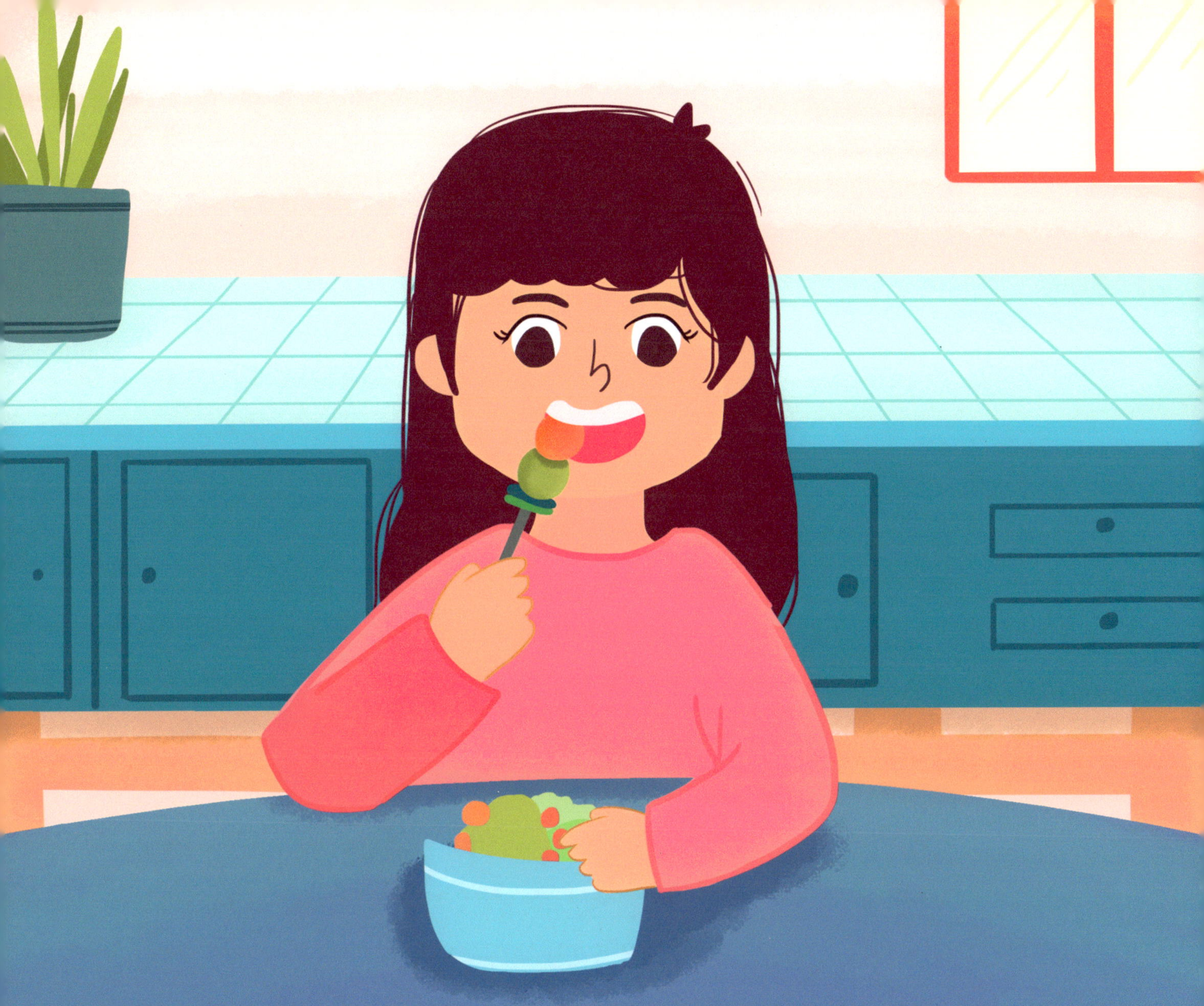

We use our **teeth** to chew food into small pieces that we can swallow. Nom nom!

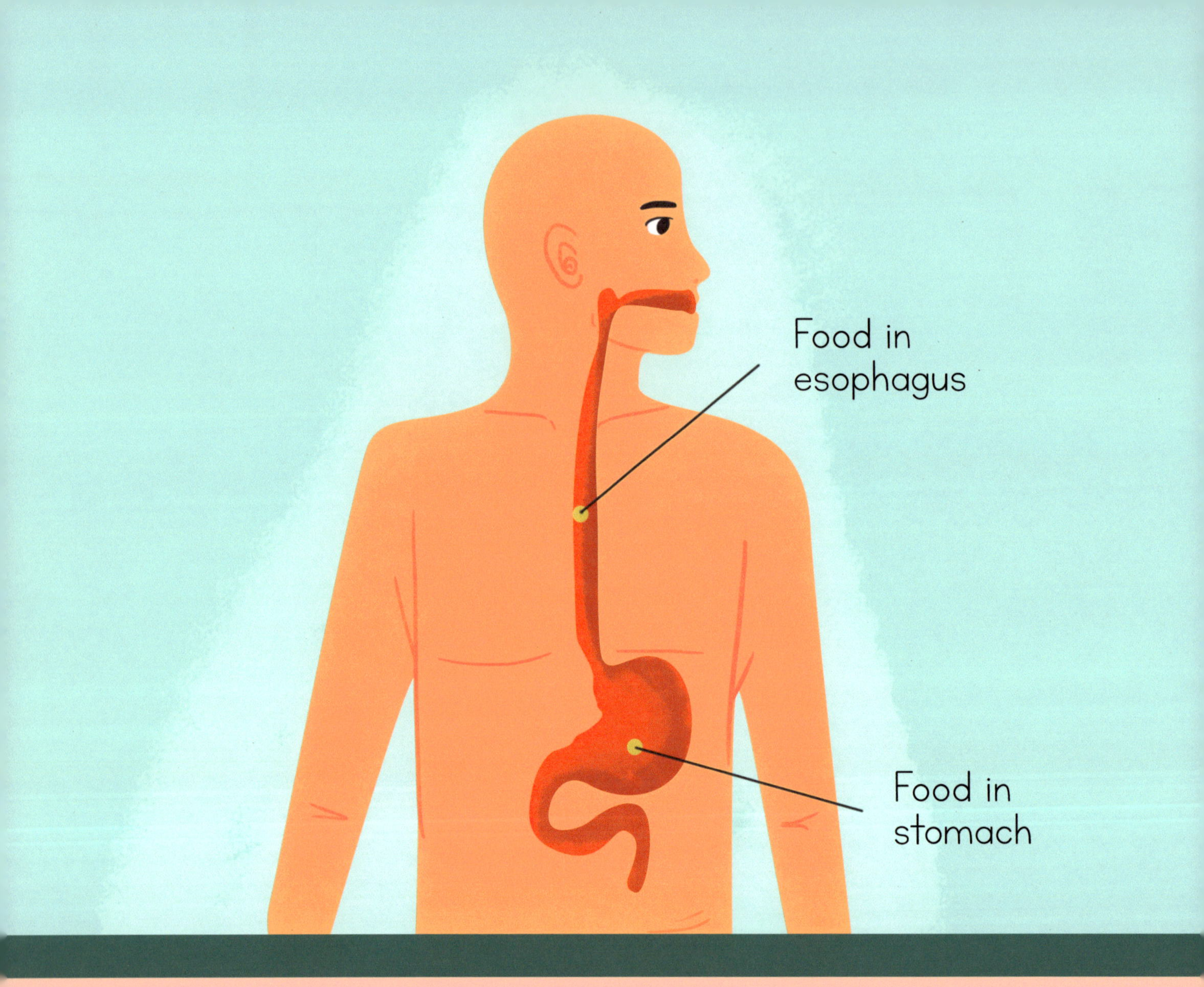

When we swallow, food goes down a hollow tube, called the **esophagus**, into the **stomach**.

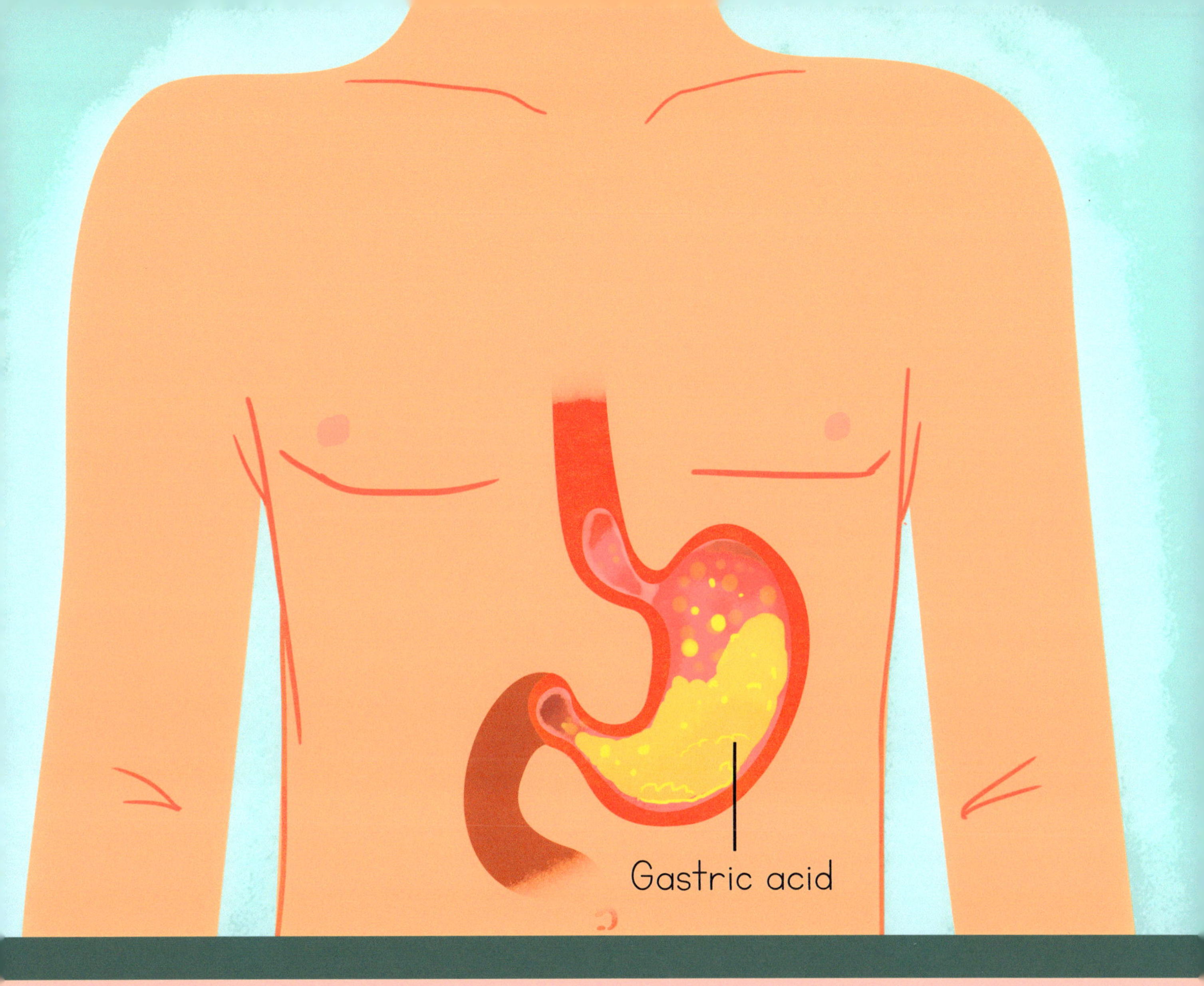

The stomach contains **gastric acid** that helps us break down our food into even smaller pieces.

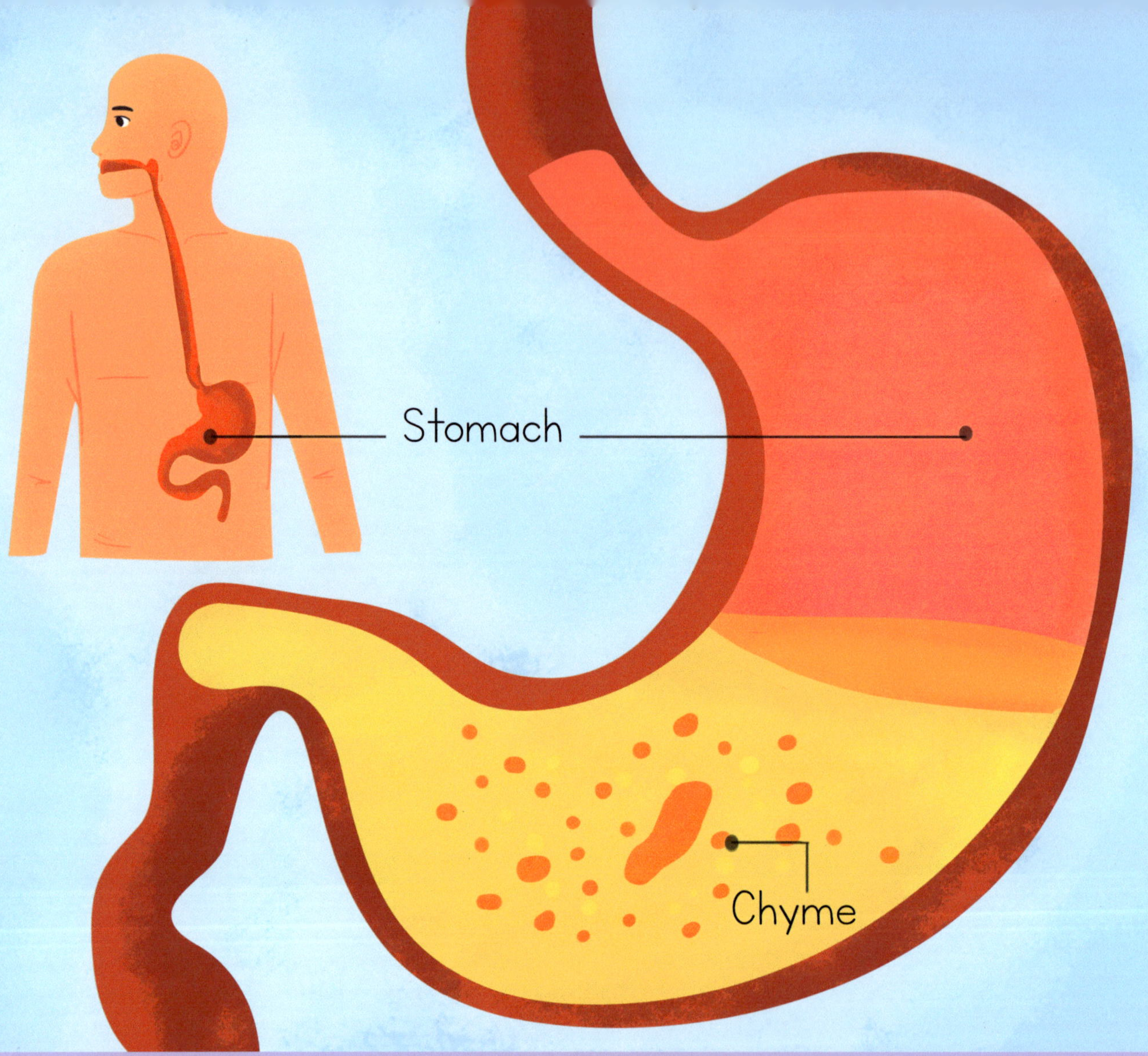

The gastric acid and tiny food pieces mix together to form **chyme**. Chyme is a mushy fluid in your stomach.

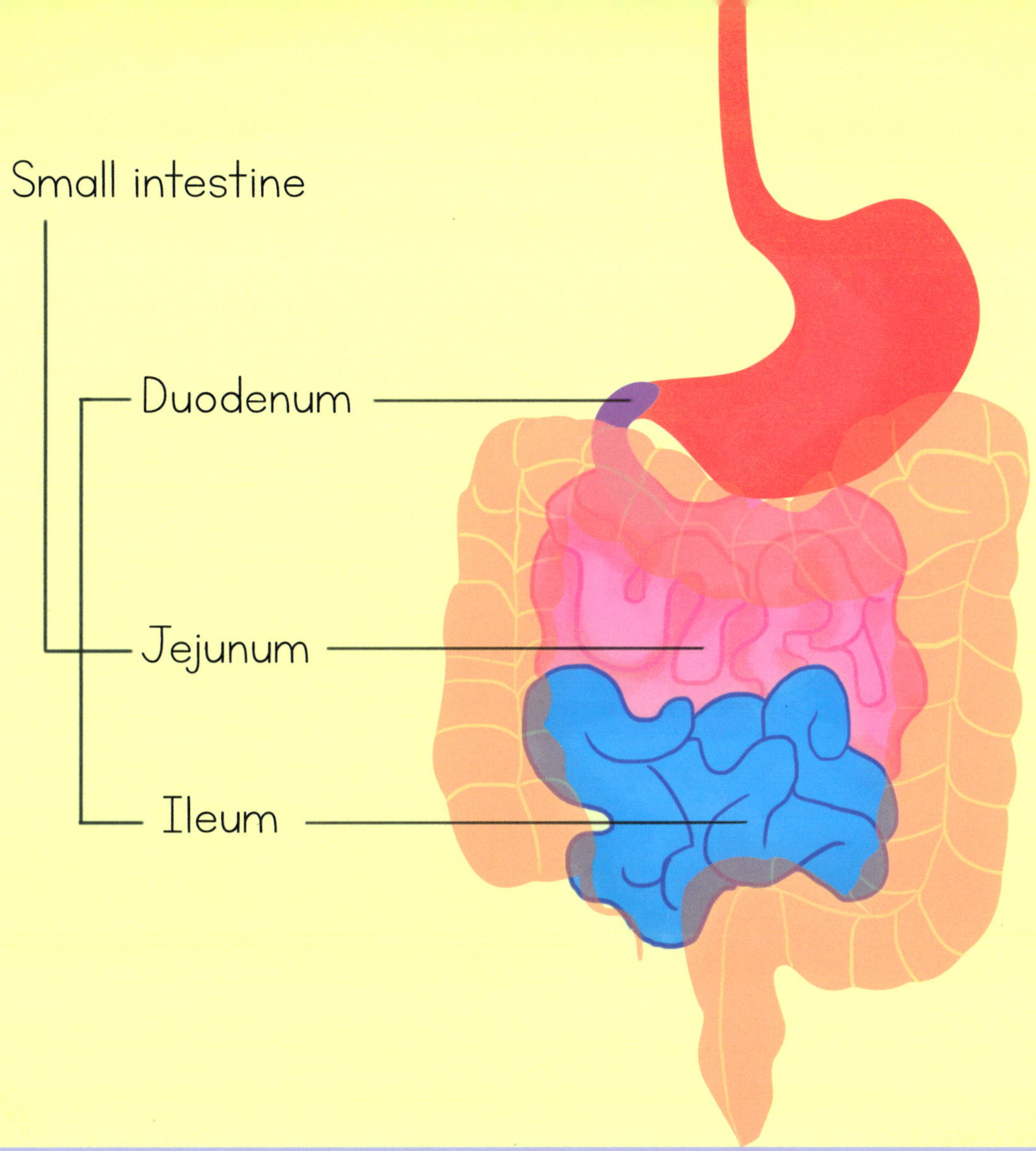

Chyme then goes into the **small intestine**, which helps you absorb nutrients from food and is made up of 3 parts.

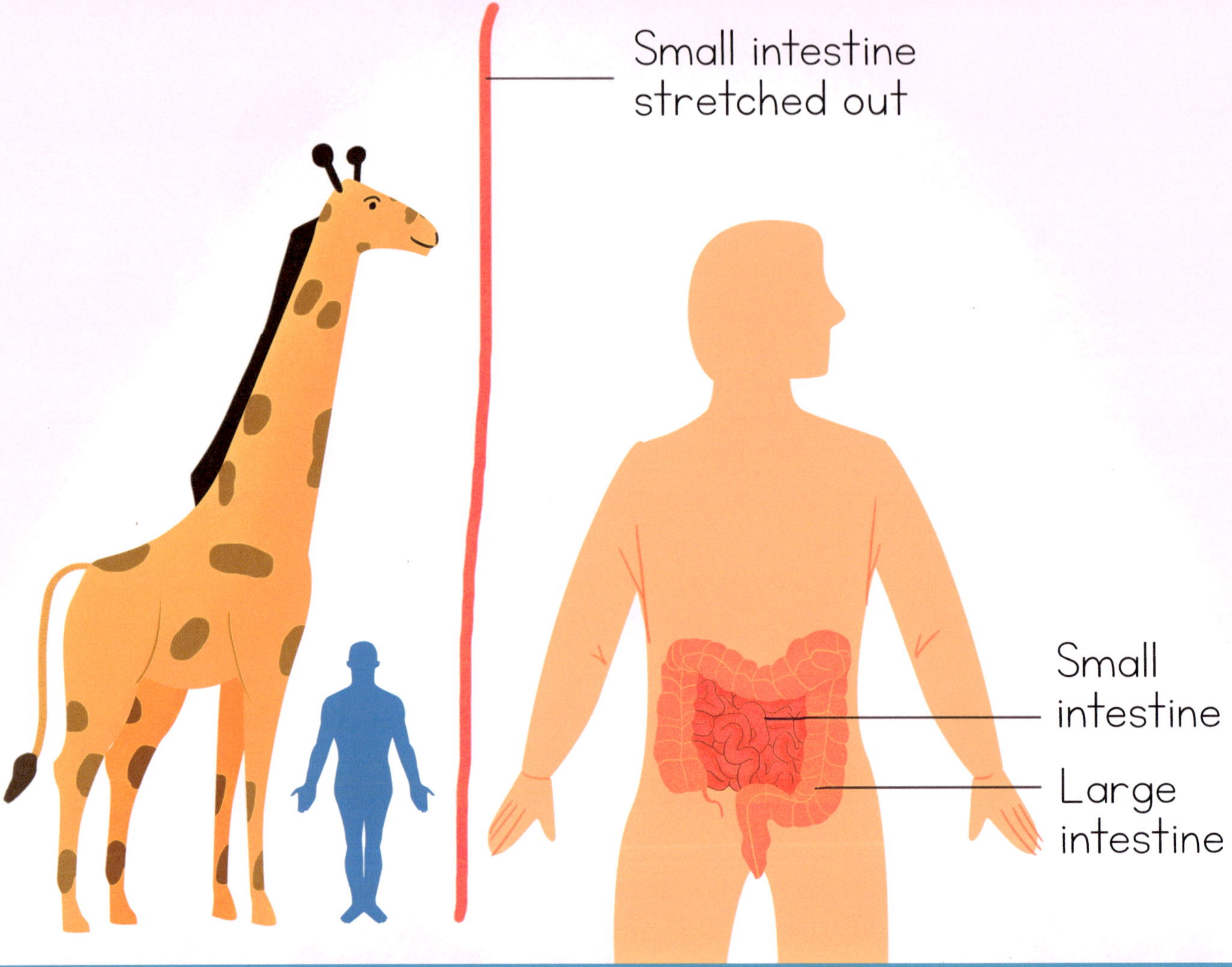

The small intestine is very *long*. If you unfolded the small intestine and stretched it out, it could be taller than a giraffe!

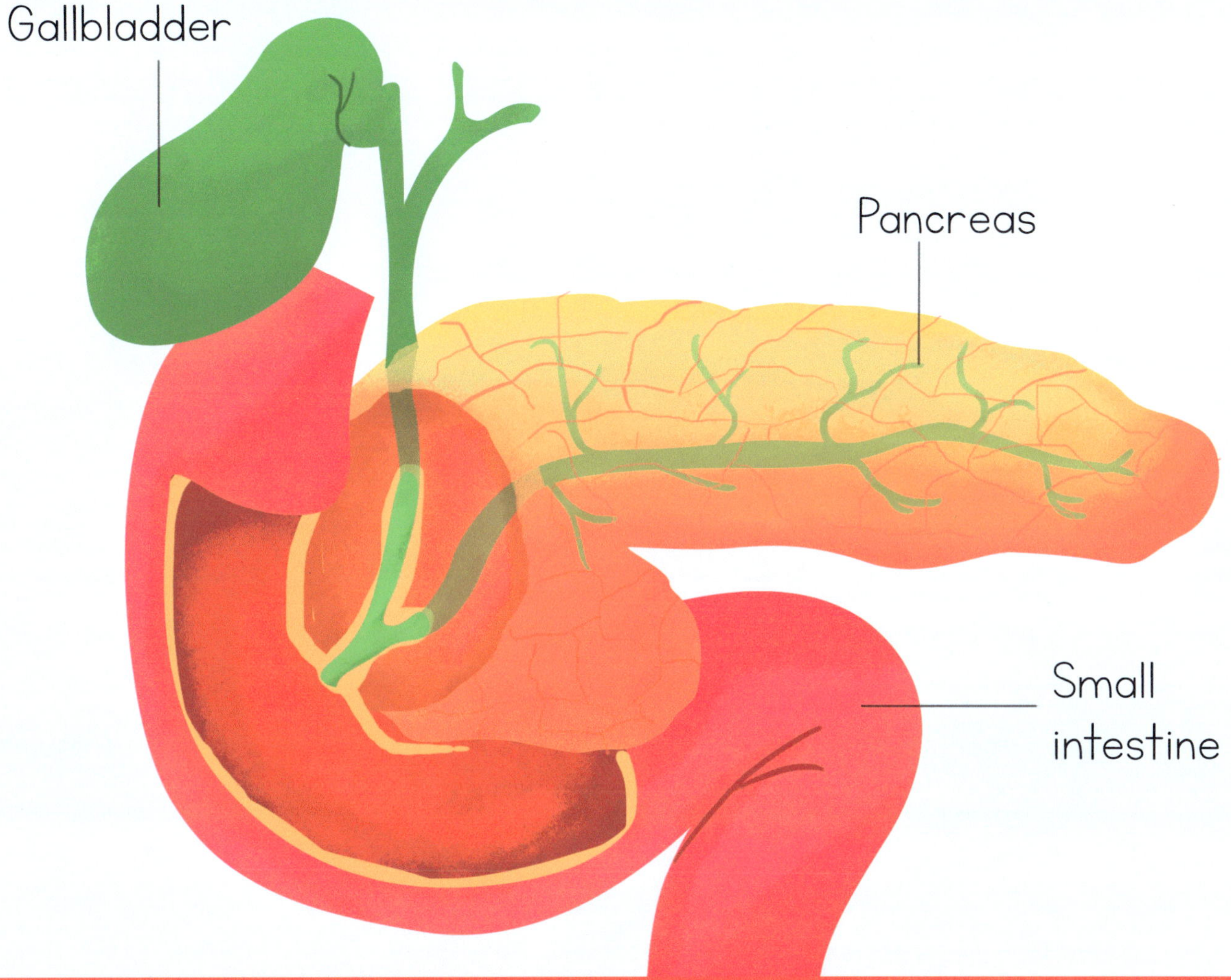

The small intestine receives *digestive enzymes* from the **pancreas** and *bile* from the **gallbladder** that help your body absorb nutrients.

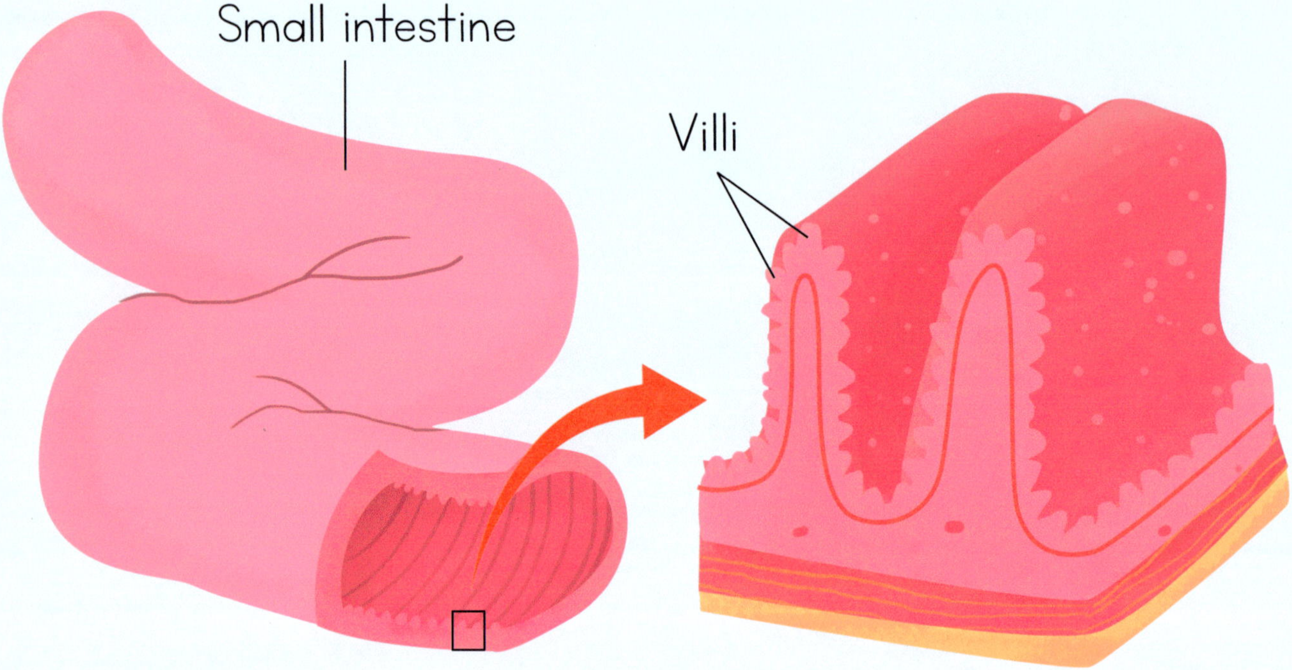

The inside of the small intestine has a lot of even tinier folds called **villi**. Villi help us absorb even more nutrients!

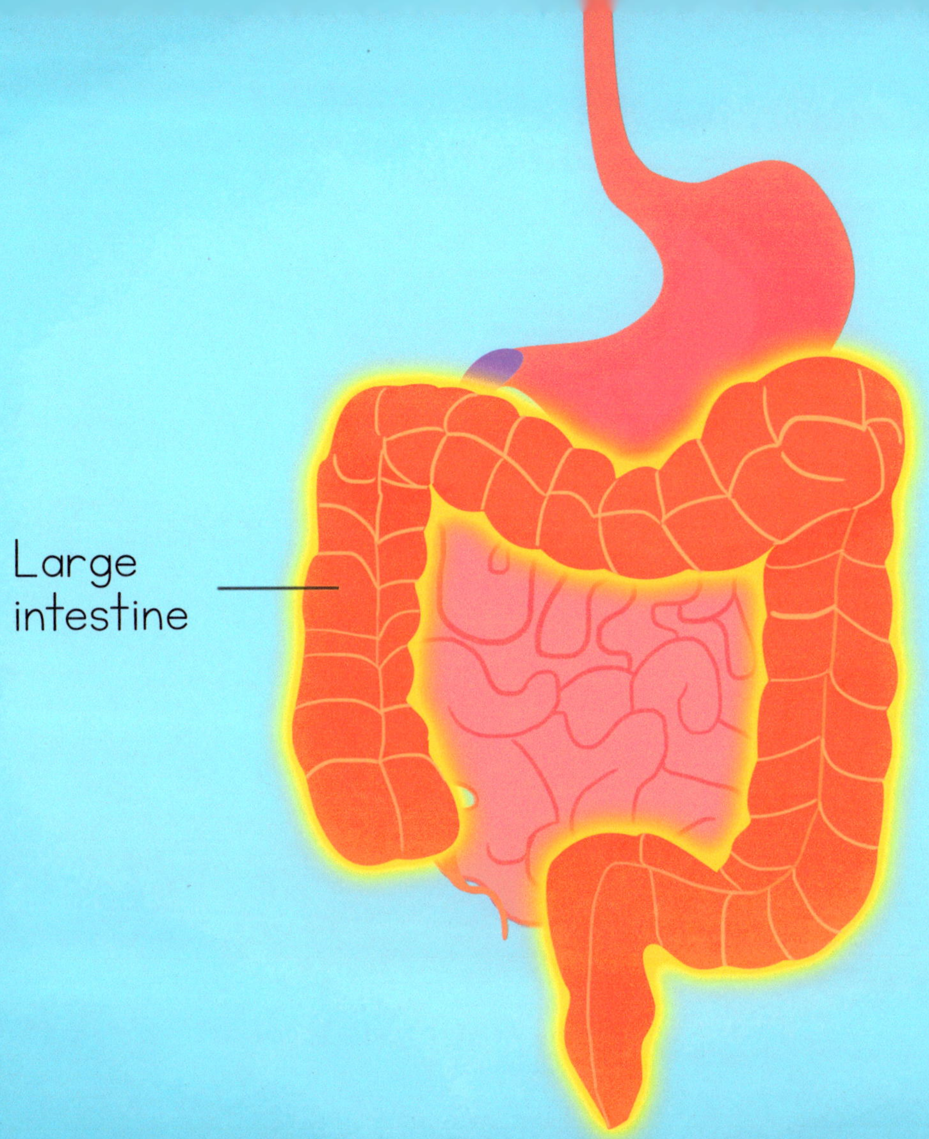

After the small intestine, food goes into the **large intestine**, which starts on the right side of the body.

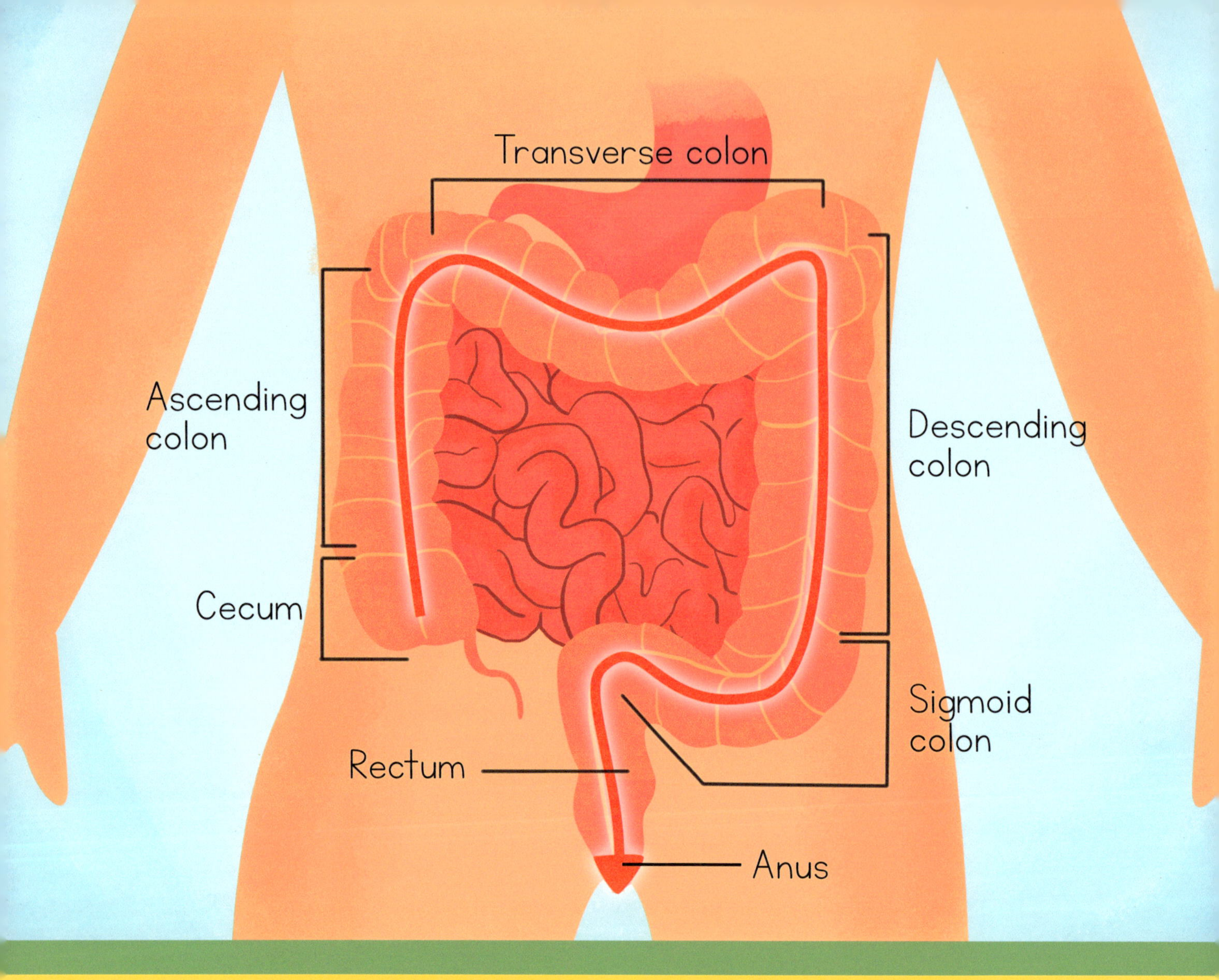

In the large intestine, food goes up... across... down... to the middle... and then out of the body through the **rectum** and **anus**.

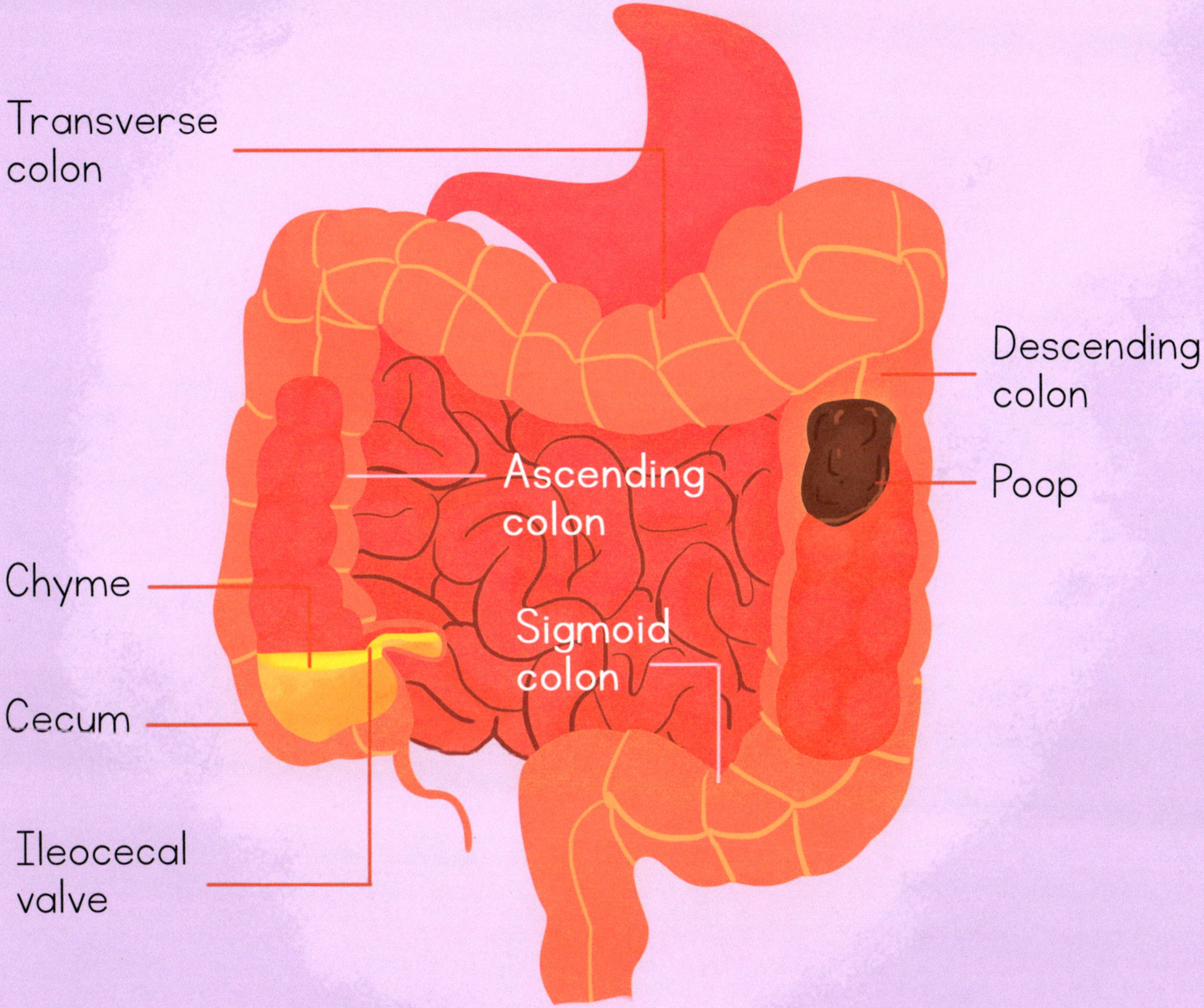

The large intestine helps you absorb water from your food. Any food that your body doesn't absorb leaves your body as **poop**!

Bristol stool chart

Type 1	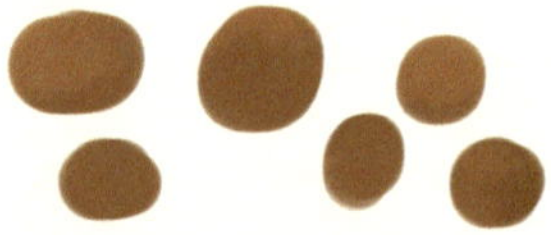	Separate hard lumps, like nuts (hard to pass)
Type 2	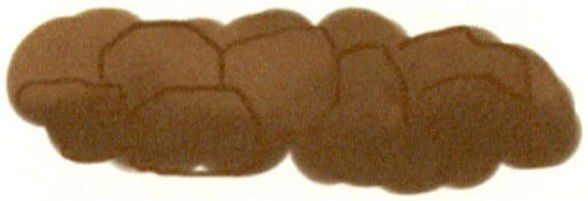	Sausage-shaped but lumpy
Type 3	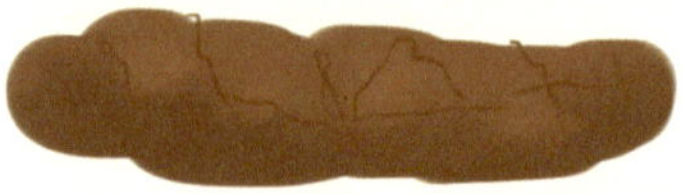	Like a sausage but with cracks on its surface

Sometimes, your poop might be too *hard*, and you might not poop for a few days. This is called **constipation**.

Bristol stool chart

Type 5	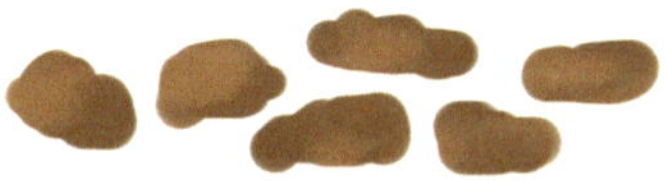	Soft blobs with clear-cut edges (passed easily)
Type 6	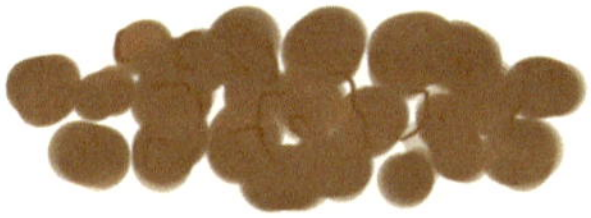	Fluffy pieces with ragged edges, a mushy stool
Type 7	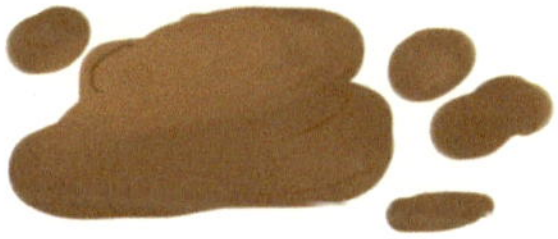	Watery, no solid pieces, entirely liquid

Other times, your poop might be too *watery*, and you might have to poop many times a day. This is called **diarrhea**.

Bristol stool chart

Type 1	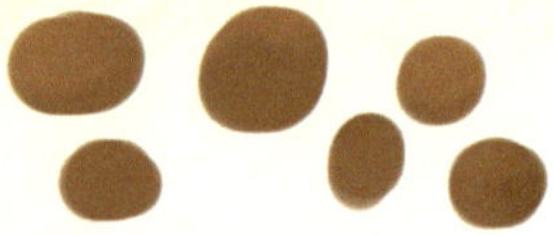	Separate hard lumps, like nuts (hard to pass)
Type 2	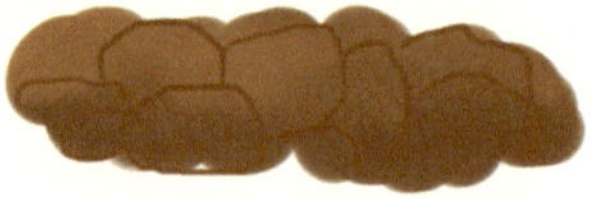	Sausage-shaped but lumpy
Type 3	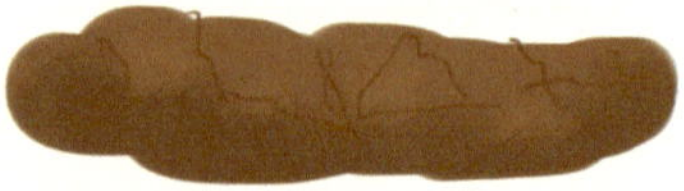	Like a sausage but with cracks on its surface
Type 4	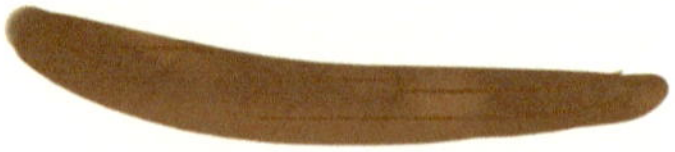	**Like a sausage or snake, smooth and soft**
Type 5	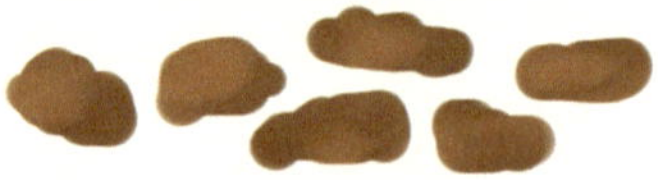	Soft blobs with clear-cut edges (passed easily)
Type 6	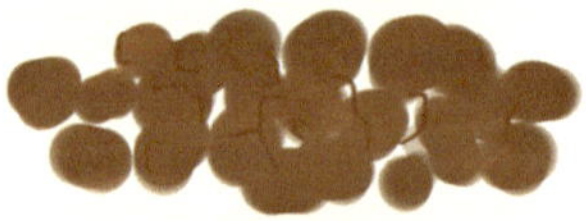	Fluffy pieces with ragged edges, a mushy stool
Type 7	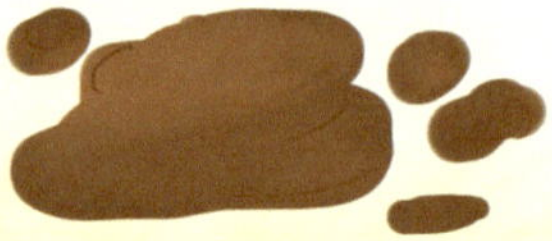	Watery, no solid pieces, entirely liquid

If your poop looks like a soft, smooth sausage, then that is the best poop!

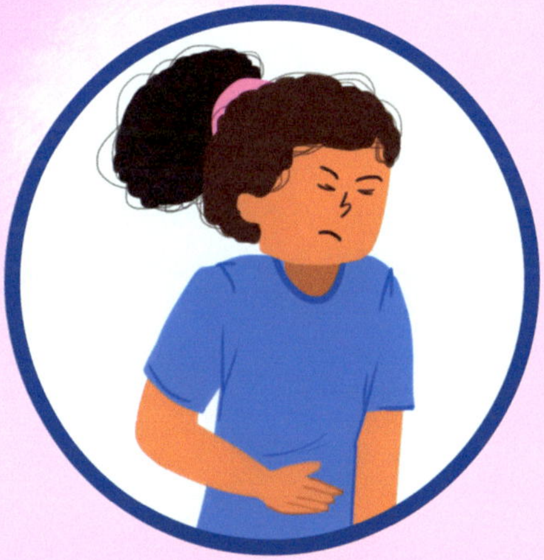

Abdominal pain

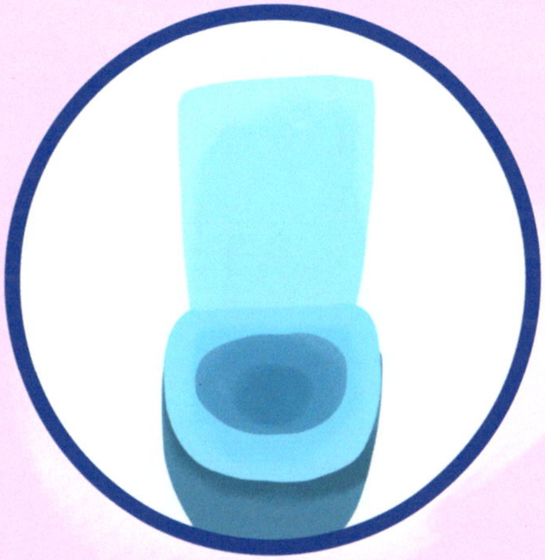

Diarrhea

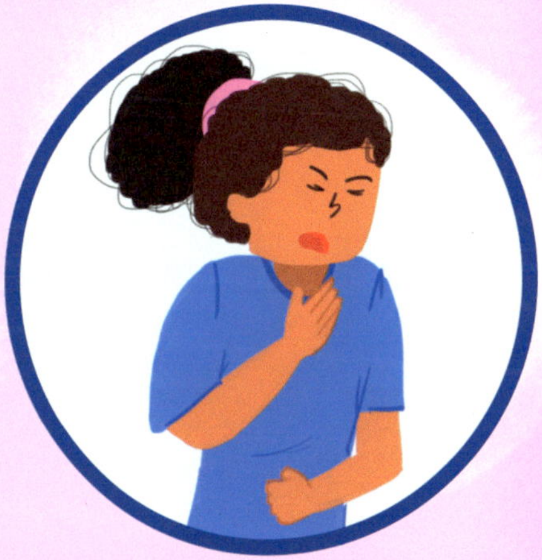

Nausea,
vomiting

Some people have problems with their digestive tract that cause symptoms such as abdominal pain, diarrhea, nausea, and vomiting.

Normal

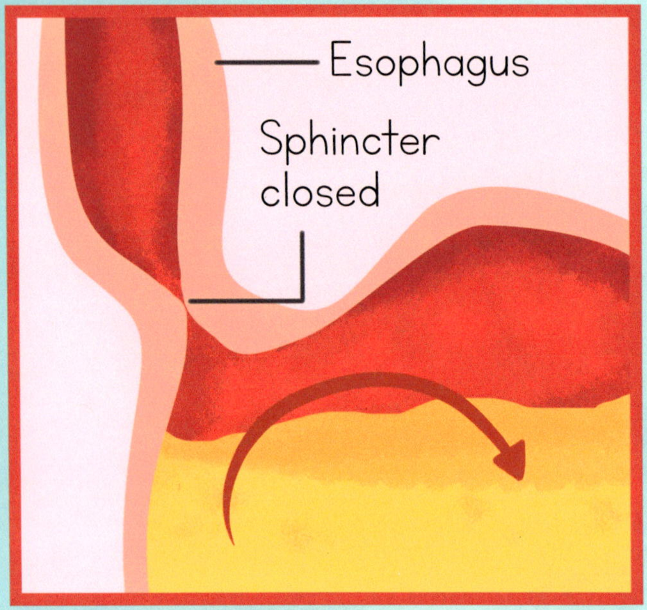

Acid reflux

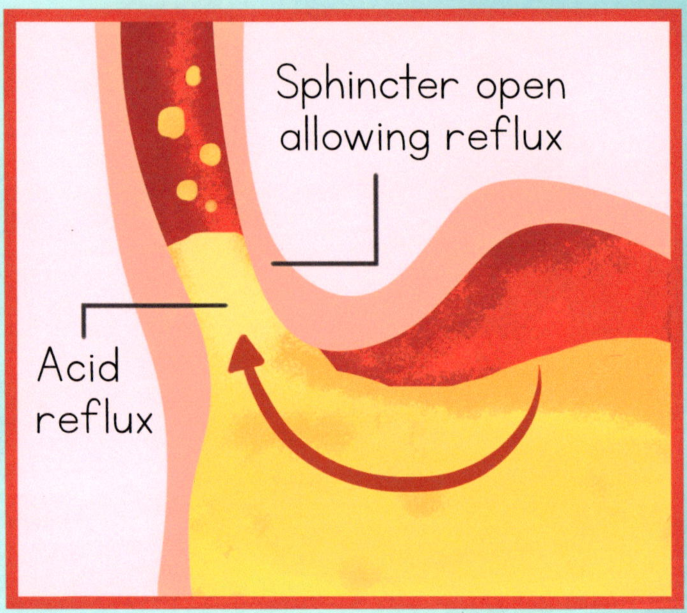

Gastric acid that abnormally flows up the esophagus can cause a burning feeling in the chest. This is called **acid reflux.**

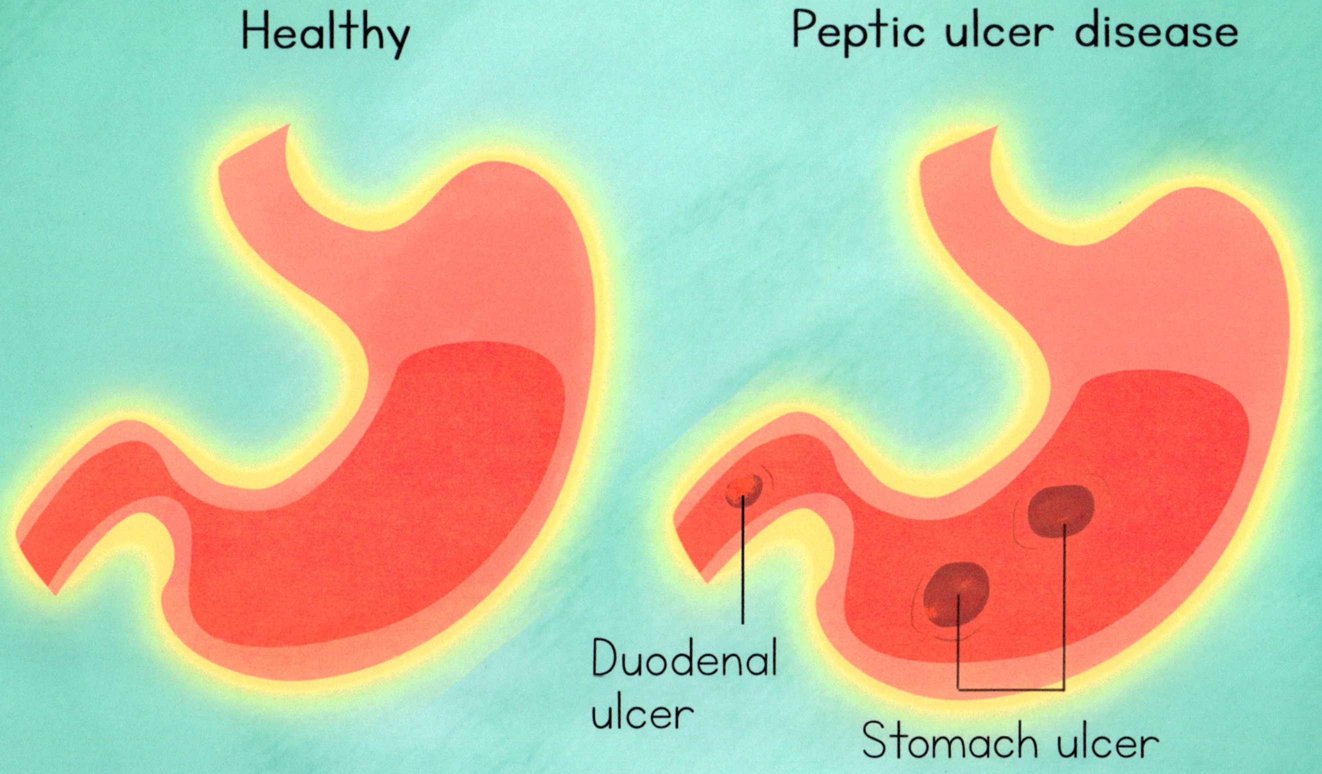

In some people, gastric acid can also eat away at the inner surface of the stomach or small intestine, causing **peptic ulcer disease.**

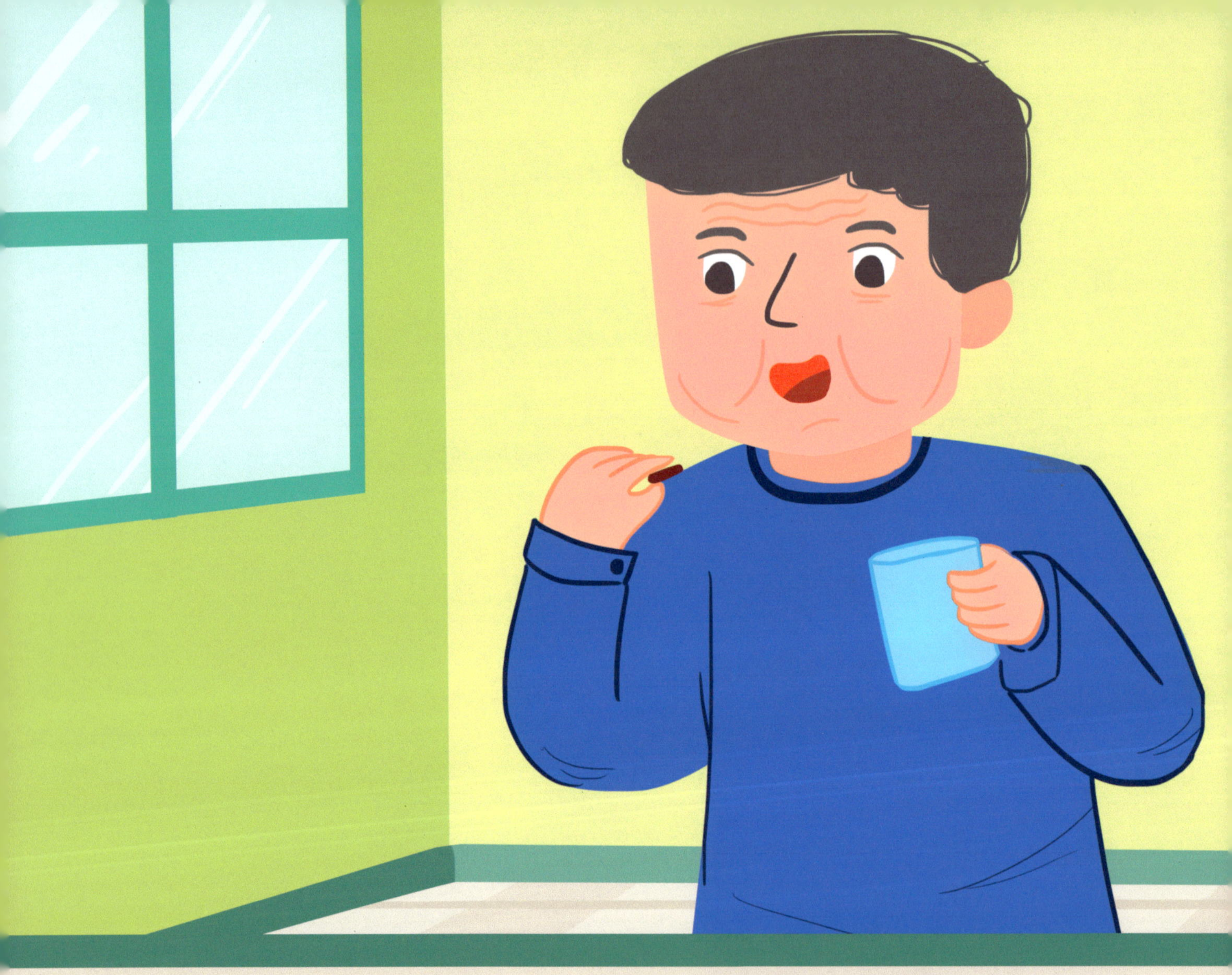

Patients with acid reflux and peptic ulcer disease can feel better by taking medications that decrease acid production in the stomach.

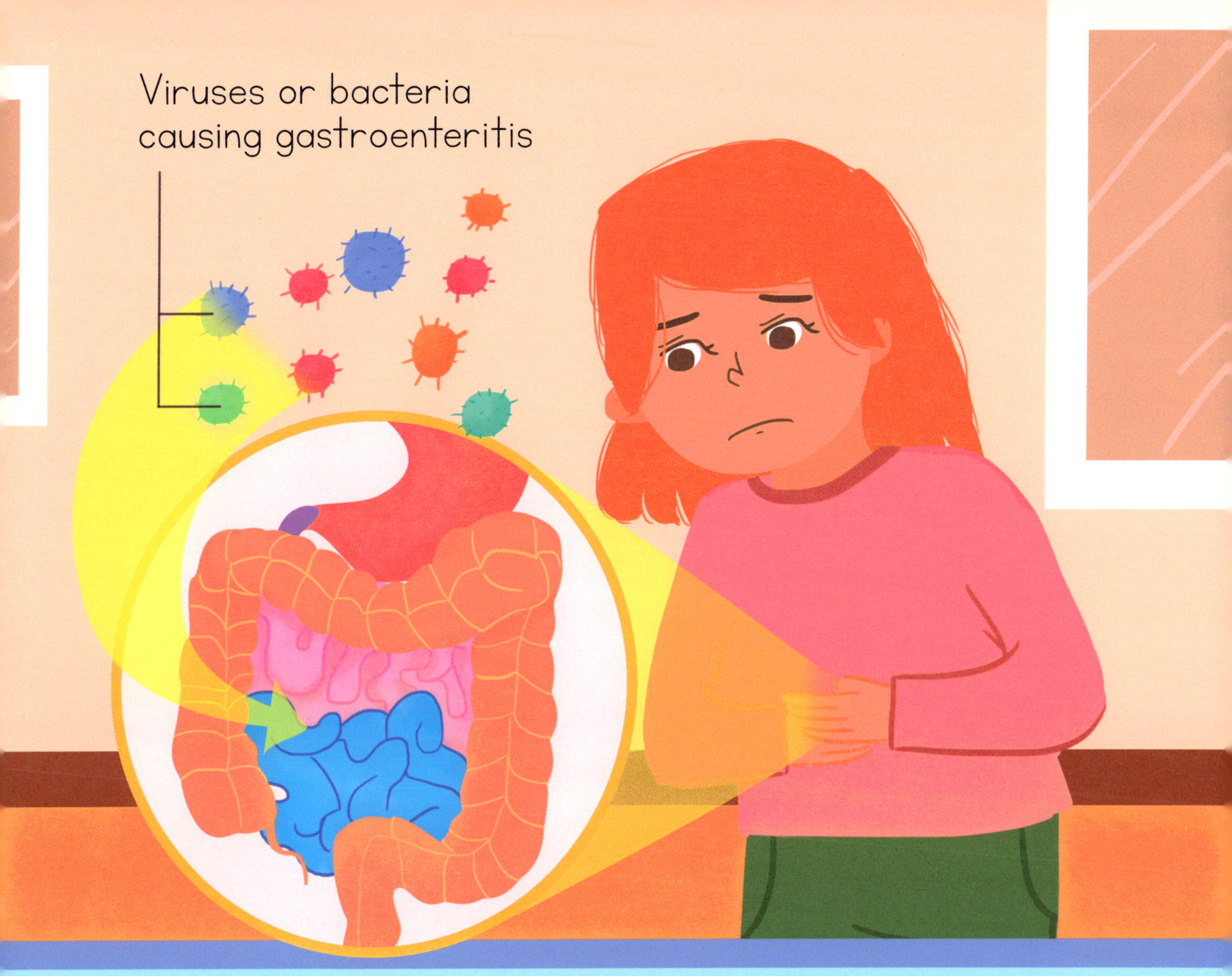

Sometimes, your digestive tract can be infected with viruses or bacteria. This is called **gastroenteritis**.

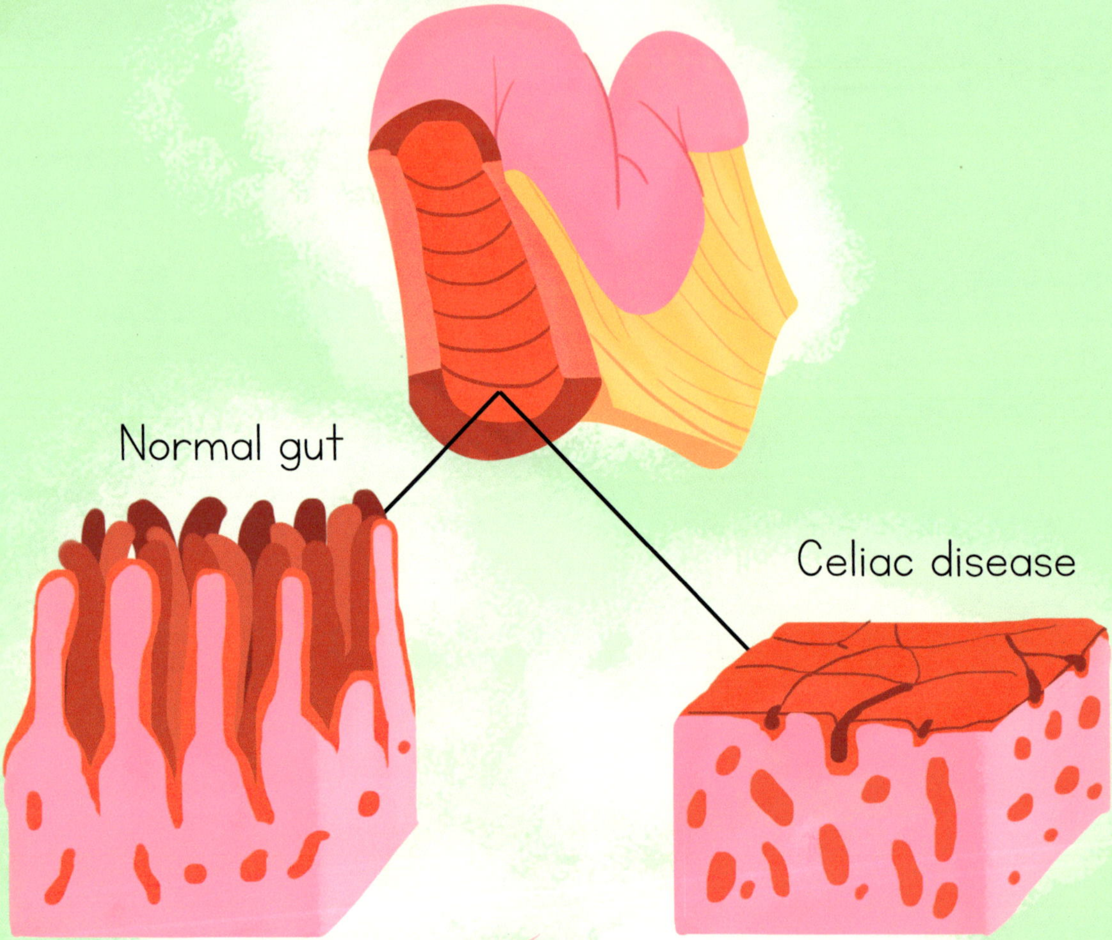

People with **celiac disease** have trouble digesting gluten, which is a protein found in foods such as breads, grains, and pastas.

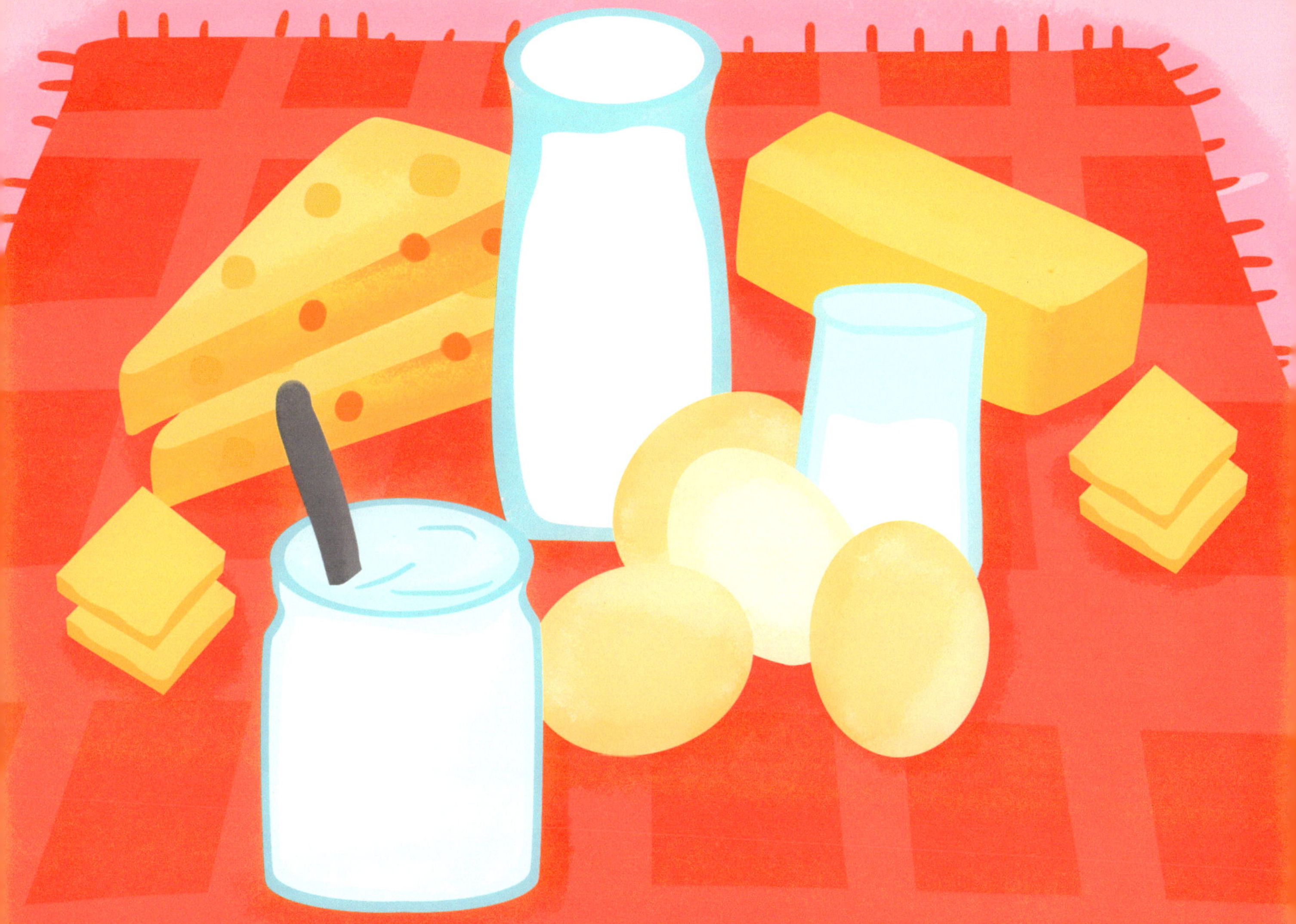

People with **lactose intolerance** have trouble digesting dairy products, such as milk, cheeses, and yogurt.

Inflammatory bowel disease

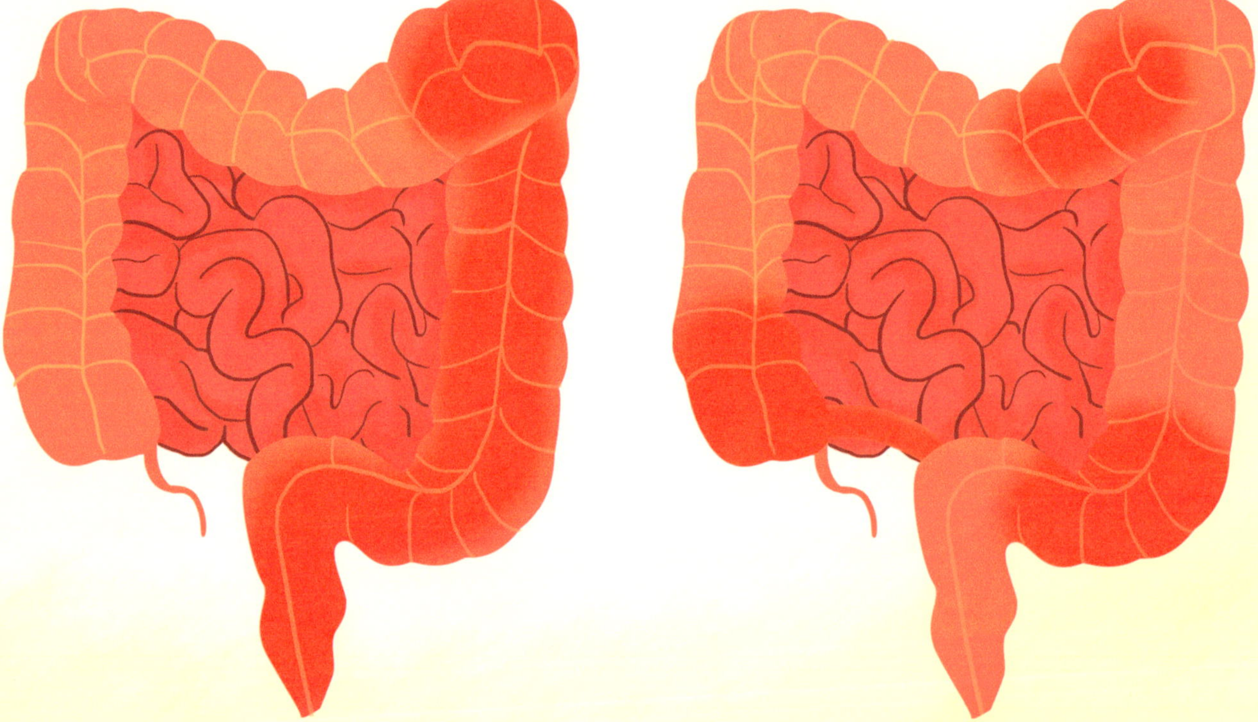

Ulcerative colitis

Crohn's disease

People with **inflammatory bowel disease** have chronic inflammation of their digestive tract. This can cause bloody diarrhea.

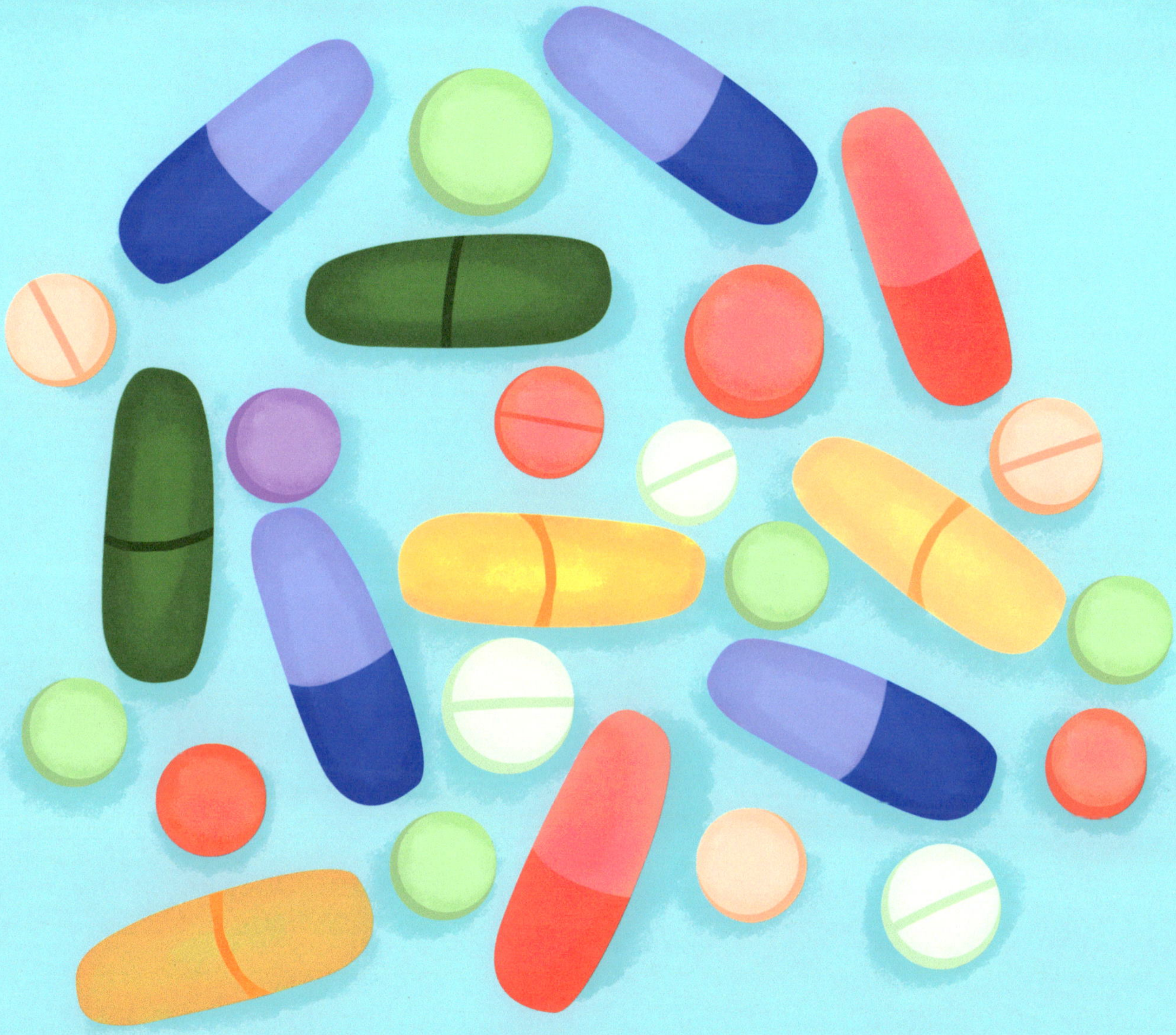

People with inflammatory bowel disease can take medications that decrease inflammation, such as steroids, to get better.

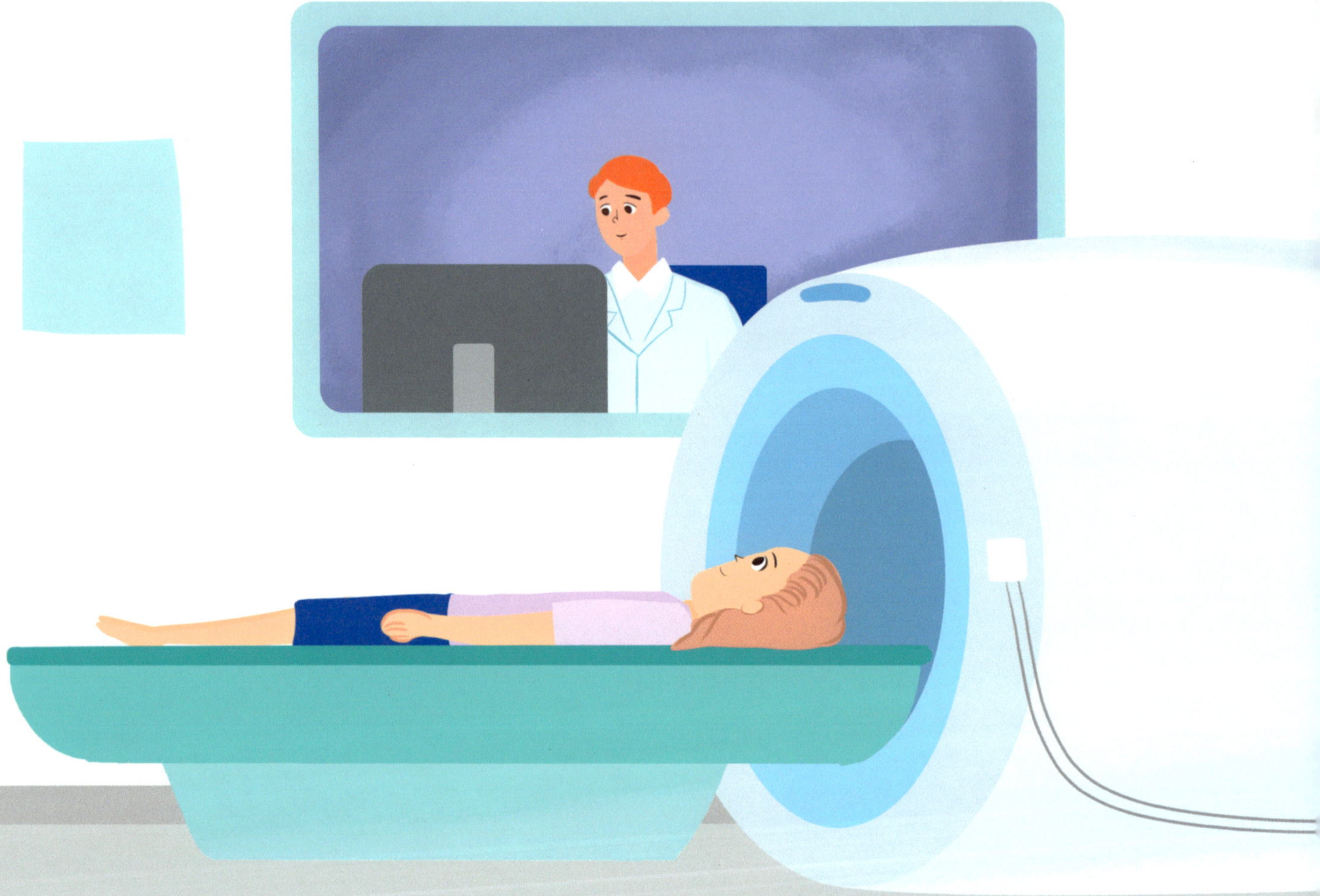

Doctors can diagnose gastrointestinal diseases using machines that take pictures of the body, such as a **CT scanner** or **MRI scanner**.

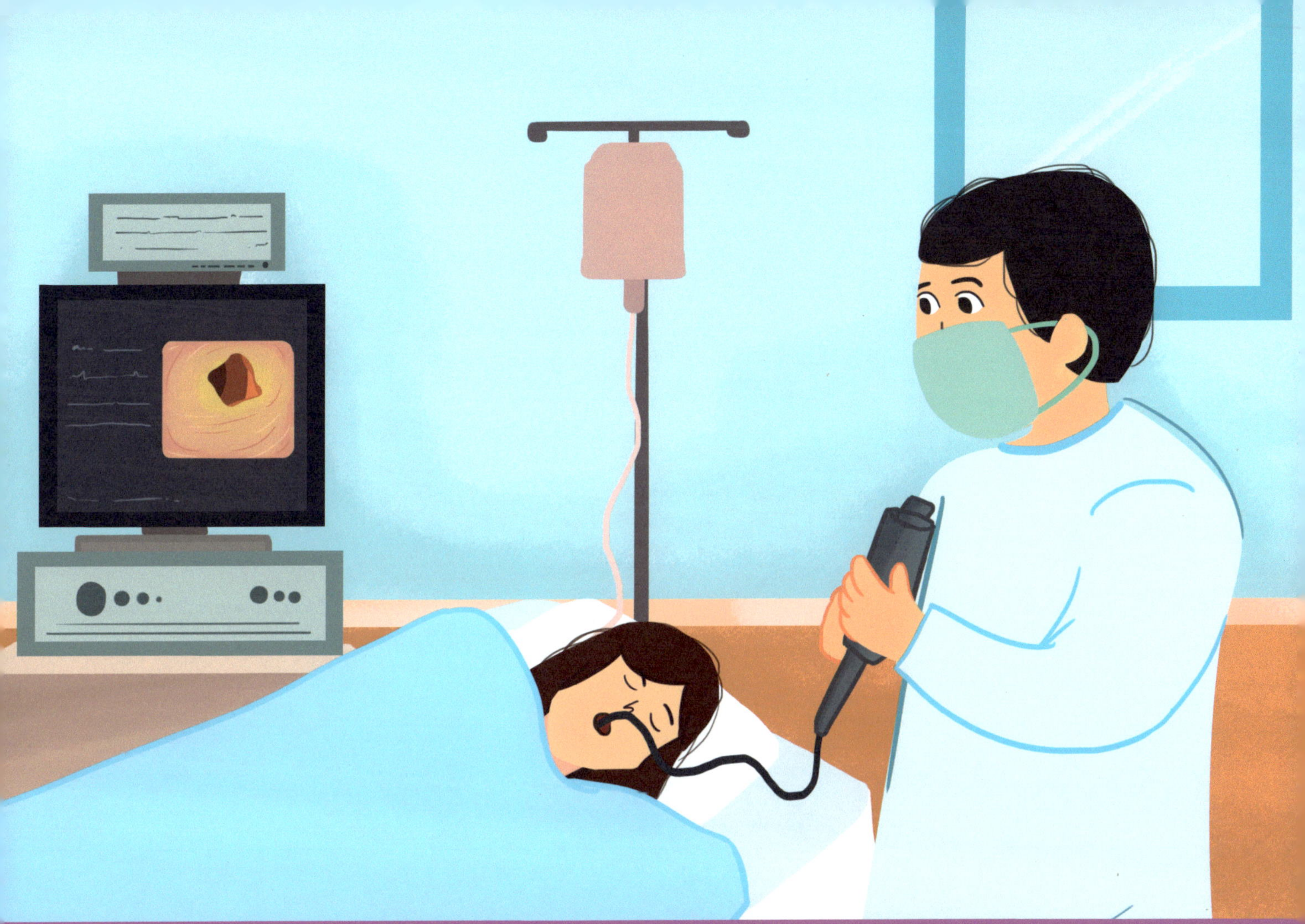

Doctors can diagnose diseases of the esophagus, stomach, and small intestine by inserting a small flexible tube with a camera through the mouth. This is called an **endoscopy**.

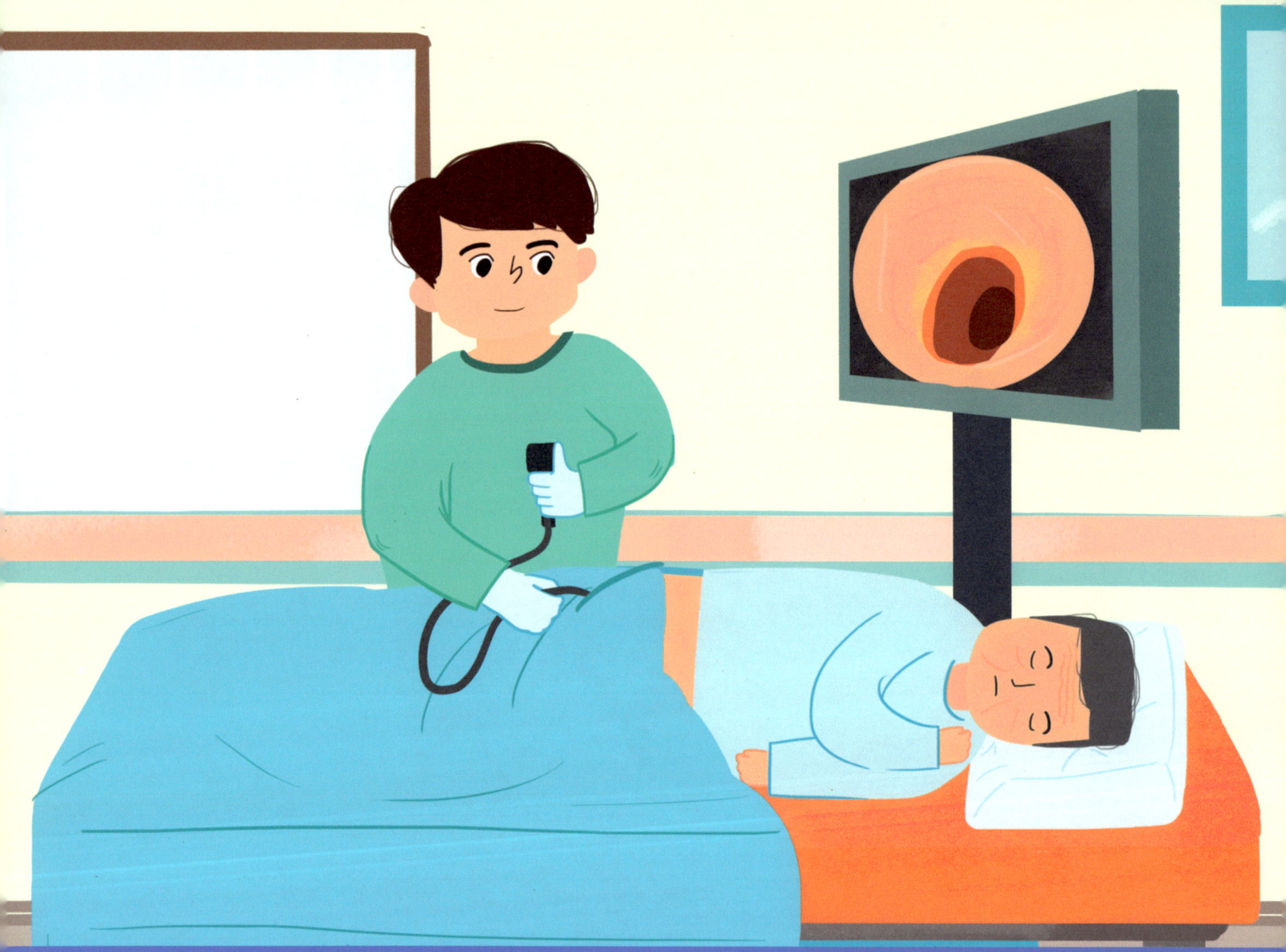

Doctors can diagnose diseases of the large intestine by inserting a small flexible tube with a camera through the anus. This is called a **colonoscopy**.

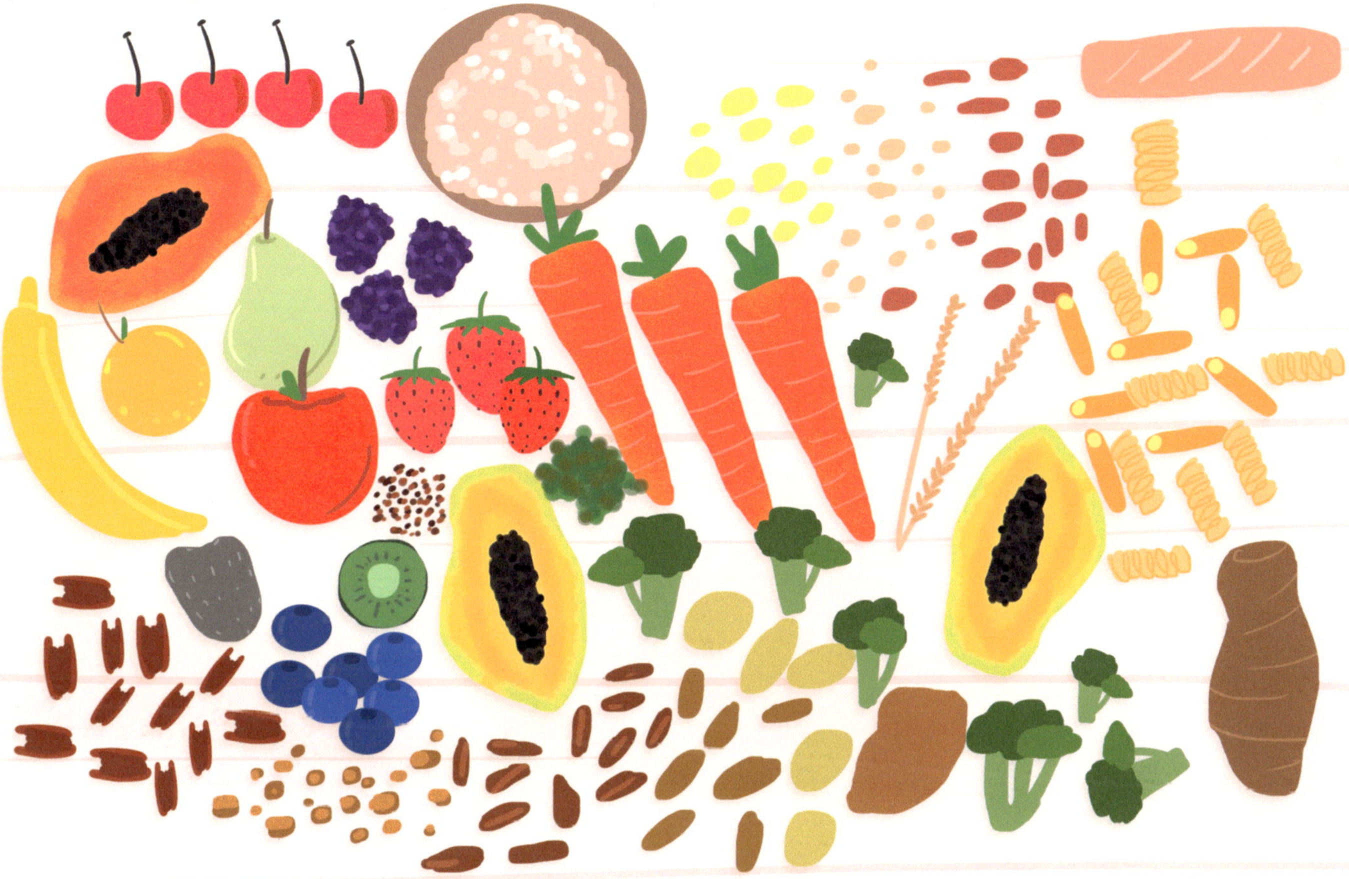

Eating a healthy diet with plenty of fruits, vegetables, and whole grains can keep your digestive system working normally.

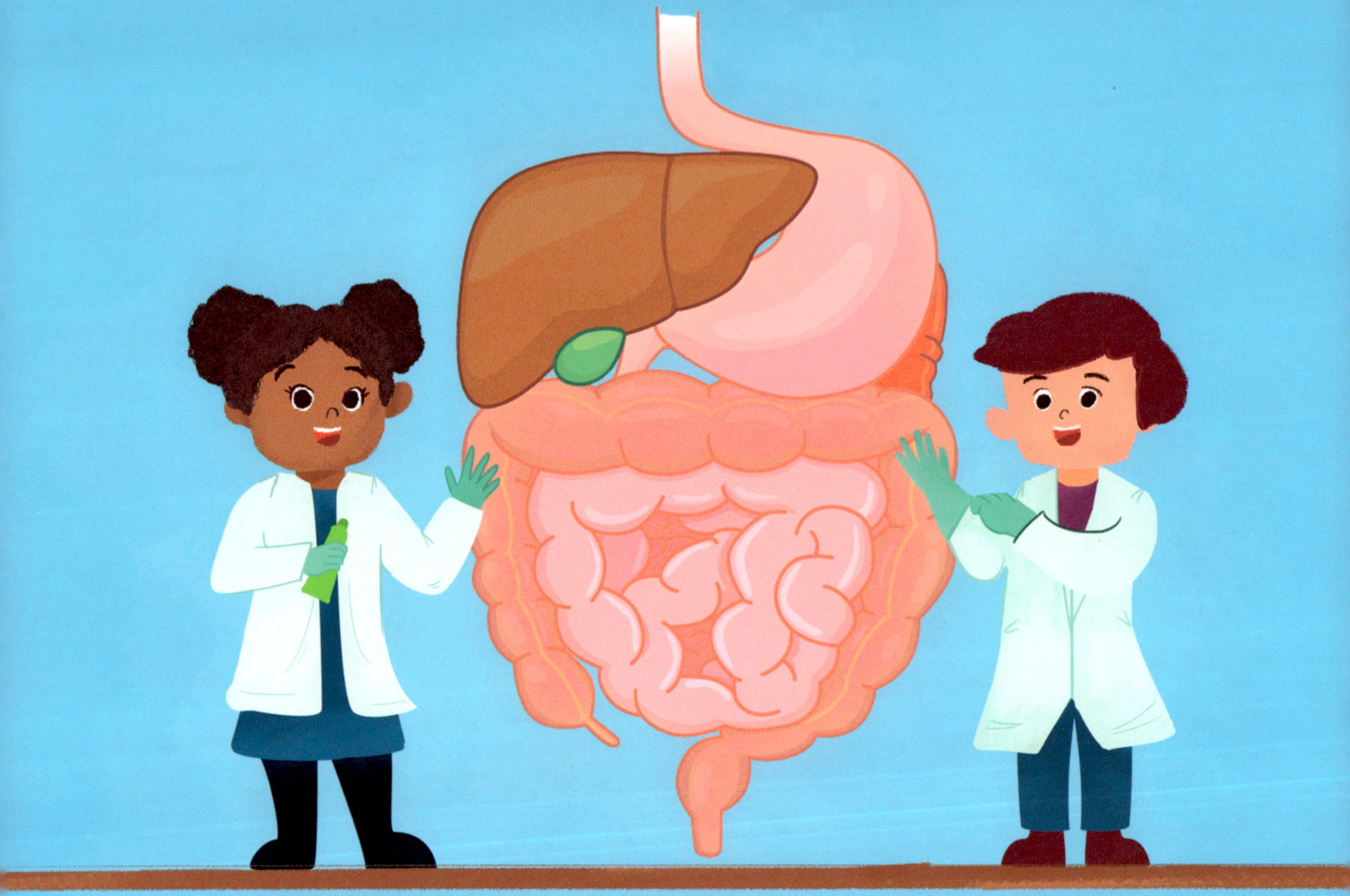

YOU'RE A FUTURE GASTROENTEROLOGIST!

Glossary

Acid reflux: condition in which gastric acid refluxes into the esophagus

Celiac disease (SEE-lee-ak): chronic digestive and immune disorder that damages the small intestine; triggered by eating foods containing gluten

Chyme (kime): mushy fluid in the stomach made of gastric acid and food pieces

Colonoscopy (kohl-luh-NAA-skuh-pee): procedure in which a flexible tube with a camera is inserted through the anus to examine the large intestine (colon)

Endoscopy (ehn-DAA-skuh-pee): procedure in which a flexible tube is inserted through the mouth to examine the esophagus, stomach, and small intestine

Esophagus (eh-SAA-fuh-guhs): hollow tube connecting the mouth to stomach

Gallbladder: small sac-shaped organ below the liver that stores bile

Gastric acid: acidic fluid secreted by the stomach that helps with digestion

Gastroenteritis (ga-strow-en-tr-AI-tuhs): infection of the digestive tract

Inflammatory bowel disease: chronic inflammatory condition of the digestive tract that can cause bloody diarrhea; treated with medications such as steroids

Intestine: lower part of digestive tract connecting stomach to anus; consists of small intestine (**duodenum**, **jejunum**, **ileum**) and large intestine (colon)

Lactose intolerance: partial or total inability to digest lactose

Pancreas: large gland that secretes digestive enzymes into the duodenum

Peptic ulcer disease: condition in which open sores (ulcers) form in the stomach or first part of the small intestine (duodenum)

Stomach: pouch between esophagus and small intestine that digests food

Let's review what you learned!

1. What is the tube that brings food from the mouth to the stomach called?
2. What substance in the stomach helps us break down food into smaller pieces?
3. Gastric acid and tiny food pieces mix together to form what?
4. What are the three parts of the small intestine called?
5. The small intestine receives enzymes and bile from what two organs?
6. What are tiny folds in the small intestine that help us absorb nutrients called?
7. Which part of the digestive tract helps us absorb water from our food?
8. Gastric acid that refluxes from the stomach into the esophagus is called?
9. Gastric acid that eats away at the inner lining of the stomach or small intestine is called?
10. What is infection of the digestive tract by a virus or bacteria called?
11. What is a chronic digestive and immune disorder that damages the small intestine and is triggered by eating foods containing gluten called?
12. What condition causes difficulty with digesting dairy products?
13. What is a chronic inflammatory condition of the digestive tract that can lead to bloody diarrhea called?
14. What two imaging studies and what two procedures can gastroenterologists perform to visualize the digestive tract?

Medical School FOR KIDS™

Your Answers

1. ____________________
2. ____________________
3. ____________________
4. ____________________
5. ____________________
6. ____________________
7. ____________________
8. ____________________
9. ____________________
10. ____________________
11. ____________________
12. ____________________
13. ____________________
14. ____________________

Medical School FOR KIDS™

Answer Key

1. Esophagus
2. Gastric acid
3. Chyme
4. Duodenum, jejunum, ileum
5. Pancreas, gallbladder
6. Villi
7. Large intestine
8. Acid reflux
9. Peptic ulcer disease
10. Gastroenteritis
11. Celiac disease
12. Lactose intolerance
13. Inflammatory bowel disease
14. CT and MRI scan; endoscopy and colonoscopy

About the Authors

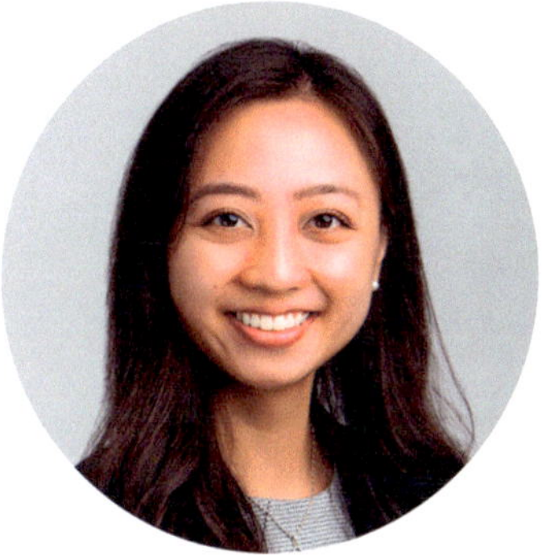

Betty Nguyen

Betty Nguyen was born in California but spent much of her childhood in Georgia, where she grew up on a chicken farm. She studied Biology at UCLA, where she received the full-ride Gates Millennium Scholarship. She also received a full-tuition scholarship to attend medical school at UC Riverside. Outside of work, she is a certified yoga instructor and licensed scuba diver. She also enjoys journalistic writing, cycling, and walking her dogs in her free time.

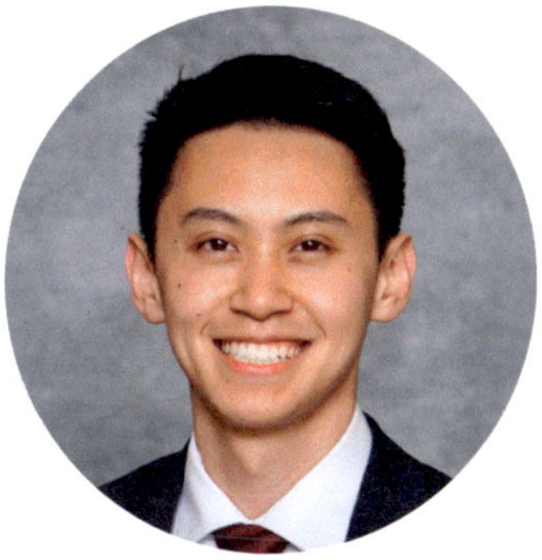

Brandon Pham

Brandon Pham was born and raised in California. He studied Microbiology, Immunology, and Molecular Genetics at UCLA and earned his MD from Stanford. He is currently completing his ophthalmology residency at the Bascom Palmer Eye Institute in Miami, Florida. He is passionate about medical education for students of all ages. In his free time, he enjoys traveling, playing tennis, and distance running.

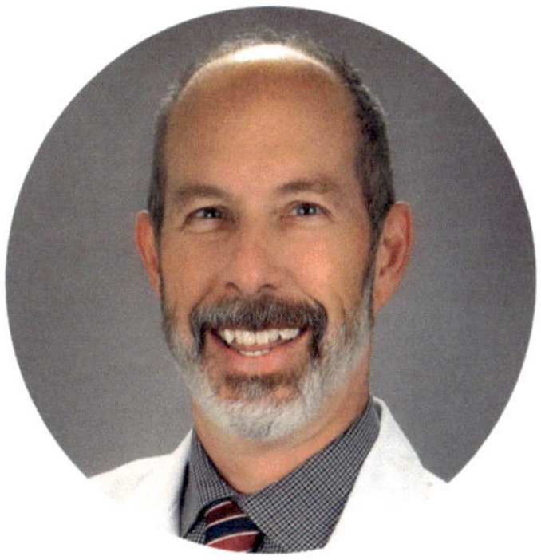

Timothy Jenkins

Timothy Jenkins was born in Louisiana and grew up in Tennessee. He received his MD from Harvard and completed his internal medicine residency and gastroenterology fellowship at Massachusetts General Hospital. Currently, he is the area medical director and chief of staff for the Kaiser Permanente San Bernardino County Service Area in California. In his free time, he enjoys distance running, biking, swimming, and hiking.

Check out the rest of the books in our series!

Website: mdforkids.org

Instagram: @md.for.kids

Medical School FOR KIDS™

Made in the USA
Las Vegas, NV
11 November 2026

57888450R00026